A CENTURY OF MAGICO-RELIGIOUS HEALING

A CENTURY OF MAGICO-RELIGIOUS HEALING:

The African, Ethiopian Case (1900-1980s)

ASSEFA BALCHA NEGWO

THE RED SEA PRESS
TRENTON | LONDON | NEW DELHI | CAPE TOWN | NAIROBI | ADDIS ABABA | ASMARA | IBADAN

AFRICA WORLD PRESS
541 West Ingham Avenue | Suite B
Trenton, New Jersey 08638

Book and cover design: Lemlem Taddese

Library of Congress Cataloging-in-Publication Data

Negwo, Assefa Balcha, author.
A century of magico-religious healing : the African, Ethiopian case
(1900-1980s) / Assefa Balcha Negwo.
p. ; cm.
Includes bibliographical references and index.
ISBN 978-1-56902-417-1 (hb) -- ISBN 978-1-56902-418-8 (pb)
I. Title. [DNLM: 1. Medicine, African Traditional--history--Ethiopia. 2. History, 20th Century--Ethiopia. 3. Spiritual Therapies--history--Ethiopia. WZ 80.5.B5]
R651
615.8'80963--dc23

2014046230

DEDICATION

This book is dedicated to my long time spiritual and intellectual mentor and instructor, the late Emeritus Professor Merid Wolde Aregay.

Contents

List of Figures

Acknowledgements

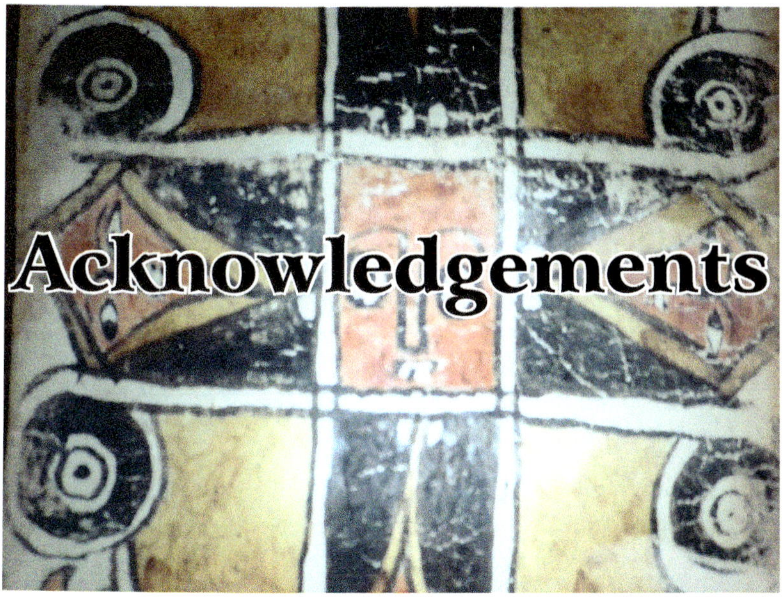

I am indebted to all oral informants cited in this work who allowed me to interview them and who candidly shared me their outstanding personal experiences as apprentices, students and practitioners of indigenous medicine. There are many others who have assisted me with valuable information and advice. This study is therefore the culmination of the inputs, advice, criticism and knowledge provided by many supportive and insightful people, whom I had the opportunity to meet and converse with on a range of original and sensitive issues. I also acknowledge the many friends and colleagues with whom I had the privilege to share, taste and refine my ideas.

I cannot sufficiently express my gratitude to my mentor the late Emeritus Professor Merid Wolde Aregay for inspiring me to work on the history of traditional medicine and for his persistent encouragement to carry on researching, resulting in this publication.

My gratitude is also directed towards Professor Randall M. Packard, at Johns Hopkins University, whose meticulous and insightful comments and guidance has been invaluable.

A special word of thanks is due to the Emory University Department of History, the Graduate School of Arts and Sciences, the Institute of African Studies and Society of Health, Culture and Disease for their financial assistance. Without the support of the university, I could not have collected the necessary data for the research.

I am equally appreciative of my Ethiopian friend and colleague, Emeritus Professor Bahru Zewde, the former faculty member of Addis Ababa University and Director of Forum for Social Science, for cheerfully reading the first drafts of the manuscript and for the encouragement he gave me.

I would also like to extend my deepest admiration and thanks to Professors Kristin Mann and Ivan Karp for reading and commenting on the manuscript.

It would be incorrect of me not to record my sincere thanks to the Prime Minister's Office and the Ministry of Health for allowing me to consult the archival materials of the former Ministry of Interior and Ministry of Public Health, respectively. I am equally mindful of the staff of the Institute of Ethiopian Studies library at Addis Ababa University for allowing me to access their rich collection of research materials and facilitating my extended reading and note taking in a caring and friendly atmosphere. At the final stages of the manuscript's production, Diana Coetzee and her editing skills were very much appreciated.

And finally special thanks to the late Emeritus Professor Donald Crummey of the University of Illinois at Urbana-Champaign who set me on the road and helped me get this important research started; and to my brothers, Kifle Balcha, Getahun Kelemu, Chanie and Samuel Kebede, and Bembela Nur Ahmed; and my wife, Genet Kebede, and my children, Elom and Lidet, for their love, and spirit of encouragement and comfort they offered me throughout the research process.

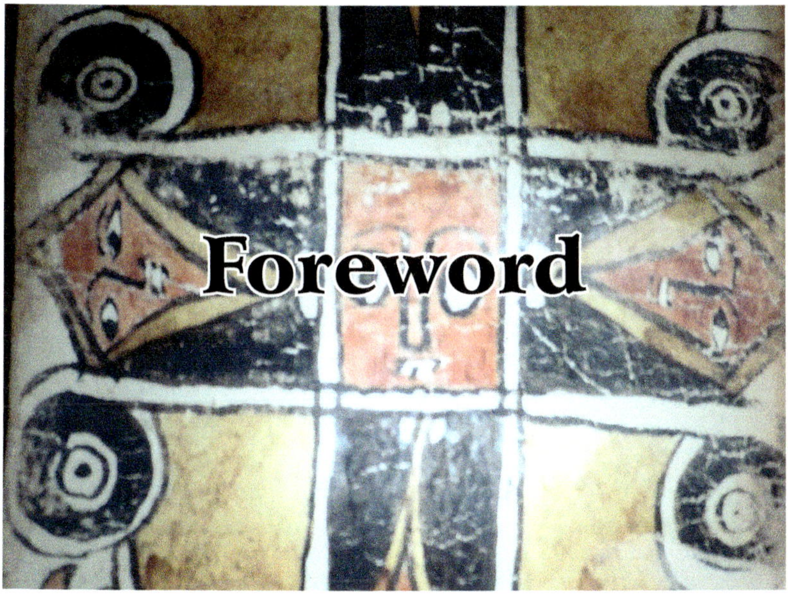

Foreword

Dr Assefa's *A Century of Magico-Religious Healing: The African, Ethiopian Case (1900-1980s)* is the first work of its kind that deals with the subject in breadth and depth. It is a very important and long overdue addition to the history of medicine.

Our reception of indigenous therapeutics is often negatively associated with our semi-feudal past, and is seen as a healing art closely associated with black magic and evil spirits.

Most of the healing practices are church-based, associated particularly with the Ethiopian Tewahido Orthodox Church. Although they are not all approved or permissible, or in line with basic church beliefs. This centuries-old tradition is deeply entrenched within the country's healthcare landscape, and is one of the crucial factors to be taken into account by policy makers. We have to re examine our perception of indigenous therapeutics and study it for what it is, its place and role in the wider cultural environment. When we have done that, we can determine how to approach the different components of this traditional healing system in line with a modern healthcare system that is being developed and expanded throughout Ethiopia.

If indigenous therapeutics are to be of any significance in the overall development of the country, they must be studied, and studied adequately. Is it possible for example, to standardize the manufacture of indigenous medicine, and if so, to make it compatible with modern scientific methods? The answer to this question clearly indicates the need for further study and research on these herbs and other healing processes and activities.

This book is an exemplary undertaking in this endeavor. It can also be included as part of a theoretical groundwork, a prelude to the actual use of indigenous therapeutics for the development of scientific knowledge.

By studying indigenous herbs that are used to make traditional medicine this sector can be made possibly as an additional base for the development of the domestic pharmaceuticals industry.

I would like to take this opportunity to express my admiration and appreciation of Dr. Assefa Balcha for this commendable work which surely required courage, dedication, perseverance and integrity. I hope this book will stimulate similar works in a wider scope and scale, and provoke and kindle a more in-depth discussion and debate regarding indigenous therapeutics at national and international levels.

Yonas Zegeye, MD
Director, The Brain and Spine Institute
West Palm Beach, Florida

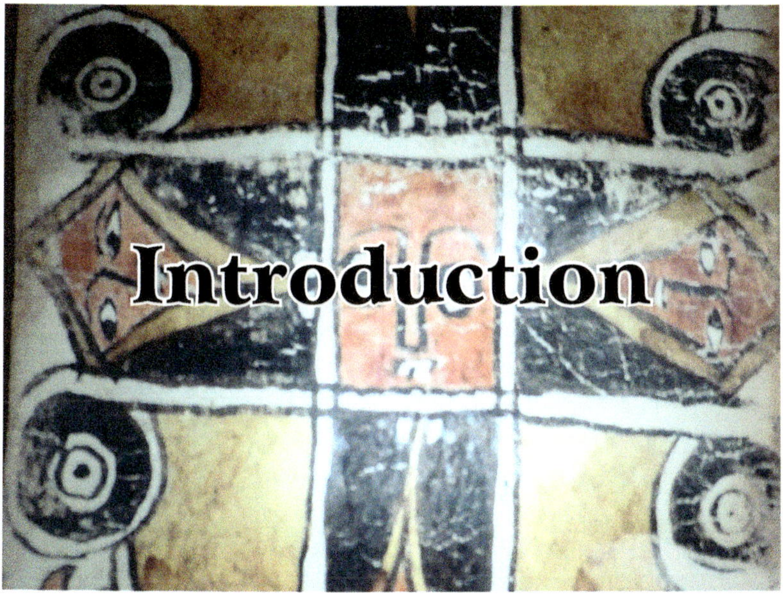

Introduction

This work seeks to explore the history of church-based healing in Ethiopia over the course of much of the twentieth century in relation to state-led efforts to control the country's medical system. In doing so, it hopes to contribute to the history of medical care in Africa, and to current efforts to develop more integrated health systems that include practitioners of both traditional and biomedicine. It examines the relationship between church-based medicine and the state in Ethiopia over the course of the 20th century. Church-based healing, associated with the Ethiopian Orthodox Church, can be traced back to the 16th century. It involved a rich complex of practices based on the use of esoteric medical and divinatory texts and the manipulation of letters and numbers, as well as invocation of spirits, and the use of herbal therapies. Church-based healers underwent rigorous training lasting many years and dealt with a range of physical and social problems. During the 20th century, church-based healers had to contend with a rapidly changing social and political environment shaped by successive state-led efforts to transform Ethiopian society. These transformations, including the introduction of western education and medicine, began with the westernizing initiatives of Menelik II (1889-1913), and continued through successive post-Menelik governments, including the five year Italian colonial rule, the restored Ethiopian monarchy under Haile Selassie and the coming to power of a Marxist military regime in the 1970s. The book investigates how church-based medico-magical healers struggled to maintain their medical traditions in the face of these transformations. Understanding the history of these struggles is important for current efforts to integrate traditional health practices into the Ethiopian health system. For these earlier interactions shaped the attitudes of both state health authorities and indigenous health practitioners toward one another.

The Challenge of Integration

Since the late 1970s, the World Health Organization (WHO) has recommended that practitioners of so-called traditional medicine be integrated into primary healthcare systems in Africa and elsewhere. Numerous studies have examined the integration efforts that followed this recommendation, and by the 1980s it had become evident that integration faced significant challenges.

Anthropologists working in a number of countries highlighted the functional and conceptual barriers to integration. These studies showed that in most instances the practice of integration was restricted to the incorporation of those elements of traditional medicine that were deemed to be complementary to a country's biomedical health system. Thus, the absorption of midwives into the formal healthcare system occurred with little problem, because their technical knowledge of childbirth, and maternal and childcare was comprehensible to practitioners of Western biomedicine. The transformation of midwives into so-called traditional birth attendants within health and family planning programmes became an obsession of developing nations in the 1980s and 1990s.[1] A great deal of attention was also paid to collecting information on herbal medicines. On the one hand, driven partly by the interests of pharmaceutical companies hoping to discover profitable new drugs, efforts were made to identify, categorize and test herbal therapies around the globe. On the other hand, spiritual or magico-religious aspects of healing were generally excluded from integration efforts, mainly because they were unintelligible or unacceptable to practitioners of biomedicine.[2] However, attempts to separate the 'empirical' from the 'spiritual' were 'bound to result not in the promotion of traditional medicine, but in its transformation.[3]

Stacy Pigg's study of the training of traditional birth attendants and traditional medical practitioners in Nepal demonstrated how integration efforts distorted traditional medical ideas and practices, producing new hybrid forms of healing that bore little resemblance to their original structure or content. Local medical practices were selected and rearranged in ways that produced an image of 'local tradition' that not only distorted local practices beyond recognition, but virtually insured that local ideas were 'silenced and shut out of development'.[4] The words 'traditional birth attendants' and 'traditional medical practitioners' encapsulated 'numerous acts of translation' through which diverse local practices were subsumed into an overarching development framework.

Green and Makhubu, examining the potential for integrating traditional healers in Swaziland, concluded that rejecting the spiritual bases of traditional medical practices would fundamentally transform healers, turning them into 'paraprofessionals' or 'second-rate paramedics' who would cease to function within the local setting: 'Such an outcome could be disruptive in multiple ways, including the undermining of a community's capacity to solve its own health problems.'[5]

It is clear that ministries of health, run by biomedical practitioners, were reluctant to move beyond a kind of token integration that failed to take seriously the ideas and practices of traditional medical practitioners. This resistance meant that in many instances, integration efforts did little more than 'pay lip service' to the WHO's primary health care strategy,[6] creating 'token departments of traditional medicine'[7] or 'renaming existing services to conform to the rhetoric of [public health care] PHC'.[8]

In many cases government policy statements were simply intended 'to please international donors';[9] and many of them encouraged coexistence rather than integration.[10] Scholars such as Komla Tsey and Daniel Offiong favoured this type of co-operation, and cautioned against the danger of venturing into integration[11] without sufficient understanding of the 'contexts in which the knowledge and practice of traditional medicine are currently reproduced, let alone the social, economic and cultural factors that determine consumer choices.'[12] Offiong argued that in Nigeria, where objections to integration have been strong, 'outright integration would be too ambitious and practically impossible, but that some form of co-operation is possible'.[13] As a consequence of this kind of resistance to integration, 'there is hardly any example of real collaboration and exchange between modern and traditional medicine'.[14]

Given the difficulties involved in integrating traditional healers into biomedically based primary health systems, it may well be that the best one can hope for is a form of co-operation that will permit all available health resources to be maximised. At one level, individual health seekers believe that they are maximising the various resources available to them in a pluralistic medical setting, moving among the various forms of healing, from government clinics, to herbalists to diviners and spirit mediums.[15] Yet many would argue that the choices patients make do not always lead to maximisation of the therapeutic options available to them. Thus, for example, those combating malaria in western Kenya note that local understandings of the causes of severe fevers, combined with extreme headaches, in young children lead parents to seek out local healers, preventing them from seeking biomedical treatment which would save their lives.[16] For co-operation to occur, various medical providers need to work together to define optimal courses of treatment for various illnesses. Given the competitive nature of the medical marketplace and disagreements among different groups of healers about the relative value of their treatments, this kind of co-operation is difficult to achieve. In addition, efforts to develop co-operation between traditional healers and biomedical practitioners needs to overcome impediments created by a longer history of interaction between these two groups.

What is often missed by those seeking to develop co-operation between traditional healers and biomedical practitioners is that in many parts of the world current integration efforts are part of a much longer history of state-led efforts to manage the activities of traditional healers. These efforts have ranged from early attempts at co-operation, to all-out attacks on the existence of traditional healers. Together, these actions have shaped indigenous health practices and affected the perspectives that indigenous health practitioners have on contemporary integration efforts. While a number of studies have described aspects of these earlier approaches,[17] none has systematically traced their history over an extended period. It is with this task in mind that the current study examines the history of traditional medicine in Ethiopia, and its relationship to government efforts to manage traditional medicine over the course of the twentieth century.[18]

Specifically, this book examines the changing role of church-based medicine in the Amhara region of Ethiopia over the course of most of the twentieth century.[19] Church-based healing, associated with the Orthodox Ethiopian Church, can be traced back to the sixteenth century. It involved a rich complex of practices based on the use of esoteric medical texts, the manipulation of letters and numbers, the invocation of spirits, and the use of herbal remedies. Church-based healers underwent rigorous training lasting many years, and dealt with a wide range of physical and social problems.

During the twentieth century, church-based healers had to contend with a rapidly changing social and political environment shaped by successive state-led efforts to transform Ethiopian society. These transformations, including attempts to transform medical care, began with the Westernising initiatives of Menelik II, and continued through successive colonial administrations, the restoration of the Ethiopian monarchy, and the coming to power of a Marxist military regime in the 1970s. This study investigates how church-based medico-magical healers struggled to maintain their medical traditions in the face of repeated attempts to control their activities and how these struggles shaped their attitudes towards integration efforts.

Methodology and Organisation of the Book

The research has made use of both oral and written sources. Interviews with knowledgeable informants provided a rich body of historical narratives. I interviewed 63 informants, of whom 48 or 76.2% were cleric healers. Informants' ages fell between early forties and early eighties.[20] The informants' personal narratives refer to different time periods and allow one to chart the changing experiences of church-based healers from the 1920s, through to the Imperial rule of Haile Selassie I (1930–1974), to the early years of the Darg (1974–1980s), a military government that lasted in 1991.

The archives of different government ministries, notably the Ministry of Health and Interior, contain correspondences with provincial and district administrative offices, municipalities, clinics, hospitals, and health, agriculture and police departments. This material provides information on the actions taken by various government departments and medical authorities in dealing with the country's health problems and with traditional medical practitioners. The archival sources help situate church-based medicine in a wider social and historical context, and provide insights into the attitudes of the Imperial and Darg regimes towards church-based healers.

In addition to oral and archival materials, the study has drawn on a wide range of published materials. Western scholars have published a number of annotations, translations and analyses of magico-medical texts.[21] Many of these scholars were linguists and ethnologists; and while they wrote little about the history of healing, their studies have preserved texts that are important for understanding church-based healing practices during the early twentieth century.[22] Some of the information recorded in the medical texts has been supplemented by the writings of foreign travellers and residents whose accounts on non-church-based medical practices go as far back as the sixteenth century.[23]

The study has also benefited from a number of more recent ethnographic studies. These studies allow an understanding of the workings of church-based medicine from the 1950s, even though these studies are not interested in tracing the history of these practices. In this regard, the research of Simon Messing, Allan Young, Mekonnen Bishaw and Dan Bauer deserve mention. They are all ethnographic and focus on therapeutics per se not on the history of practitioners and the 'professionalisation' of the traditional healing system(s).

Allan Young has made significant contributions to the understanding of the magico-medical expertise of the *dabtara* healers (itinerant religious figures) during the 1970s.[24] He described how the *dabtara* monopolised knowledge or controlled its distribution and prevented it from being disseminated beyond their ranks.[25] Young also demonstrated the limitations of the 'Western medical paradigm' to understand the persistence of indigenous healing in the Amhara society[26] by examining the social and cultural contexts of the *awda nagast* (treatise of divination) divinatory techniques and the technical operations of the *dabtara* diviner.[27]

Messing's study described the role of the *dabtara* and the different types of medical specialists providing therapeutic service in the region during the 1950s. It is principally an ethnographic narrative of the various political, economic and social structure of the Amhara of Begemder.[28] However, when linked with Young's work, it provides material for comparing changing medical practices over the second half of the twentieth century. Mekonnen's research focuses on efforts to integrate indigenous and cosmopolitan medical systems, and has been helpful in understanding more recent developments in the history of church-based healing.[29]

Dan Bauer, working among the Tigray, who share the faith of the Orthodox Church with the Amhara, has also described the work of church-based healers, called *deftera* by the people in Tigray. He explains how they were consulted and the kinds of cures they could provide in the late 1960s. He also discusses their training, though not in any depth. There is no discussion of their relation to the state and, in fact, no reference to the broader social and economic, let alone historical, contexts in which the *deftera* operated.[30]

Finally, it is important to acknowledge the contributions of historian Richard Pankhurst, who has written extensively on the history of medicine in Ethiopia. His works have been exceptionally important for their meticulous citations to historical/medical texts. However, his studies have been mostly focused on the history of epidemics and transmissible diseases, and on some descriptions of indigenous cures.[31] He has also written a great deal on the development of Western biomedicine in Ethiopia.[32] Unfortunately, he has relatively little to say about the history of church-based healing.

This work provides a brief survey of Ethiopian society at the time when some Western-oriented changes began to permeate the country. The restricted efforts of Ethiopian rulers to popularise Western education and medicine, and the challenges they posed to indigenous institutions are reviewed. The medical landscape that existed at the beginning of the twentieth century is described as one that was occupied by a wide range of healers among whom were church-based healers who occupied a dominant position in this landscape. The book looks at the training of church-based healers during the 1920s and 1930s, which provided them with privileged access to magico-medical knowledge and techniques, and supported their claims to superior medical expertise. The nature of student–teacher relationships and the methods of church-based magico-medical education at the time are also described. Religious students developed an interest in and joined selected religious institutions to learn church-based medicine. The motivational factors, recruitment procedures and educational sites are examined in this study.

Church-based healers faced many challenges, beginning in the 1930s with the Italian occupation. This study shows how this shaped their practices and attitudes towards the state. The Italian Interlude (1935/36–1941) describes the Italian colonial policy towards the Orthodox Church and church-based healers, and why the colonial officials wanted to eliminate them from the scene. This section also touches on how the Italians succeeded in beginning to popularise European biomedicine in Ethiopia.

The section on 'Biomedicine, the Bureaucracy and the Quest for Alternative Therapy (1941-1974)' explores the health policies of the restored imperial government and the manifold bureaucratic/administrative problems that beleaguered their efforts to expand the biomedical healthcare system from the end of the Italian interlude to the 1974 revolution. It also investigates how the limits of Western healthcare coverage provided space within which various forms of indigenous healing could function and for the emergence of new forms of hybrid medical care, including that provided by a growing number of so-called injectionists.

In the chapter on church-based medicine and healing in the post-Italian era the position of cleric healers during the Imperial era is discussed, with a focus on the state's efforts to legalise indigenous medicine, while at the same time supporting state structures that limited the ability of church-based healers to function freely.

The expansion of literacy through Western education, and the introduction of printing technology, which led to the publication of a number of formerly secret medical texts, challenged the authority of church-based healers, by undermining their claims to having privileged access to specialised skills and knowledge. The period 1974 to the early 1980s sees the Marxist military government's anti-religious stance and its relentless attacks on church-based healers. The book also attempts to look at how the Darg subsequently attempted to integrate indigenous healing into its primary healthcare system, while trying to strip off its religious content. These policies alienated church-based healers and, at the same time, they weakened their position in Ethiopian society. They also made healers extremely suspicious and unsupportive of any state-sponsored initiative towards indigenous medicine; attitudes that have continued up to the present, limiting efforts to develop an integrated healthcare system in Ethiopia today.

Figure 1: A personal amulet against an illness called 'Nedra'

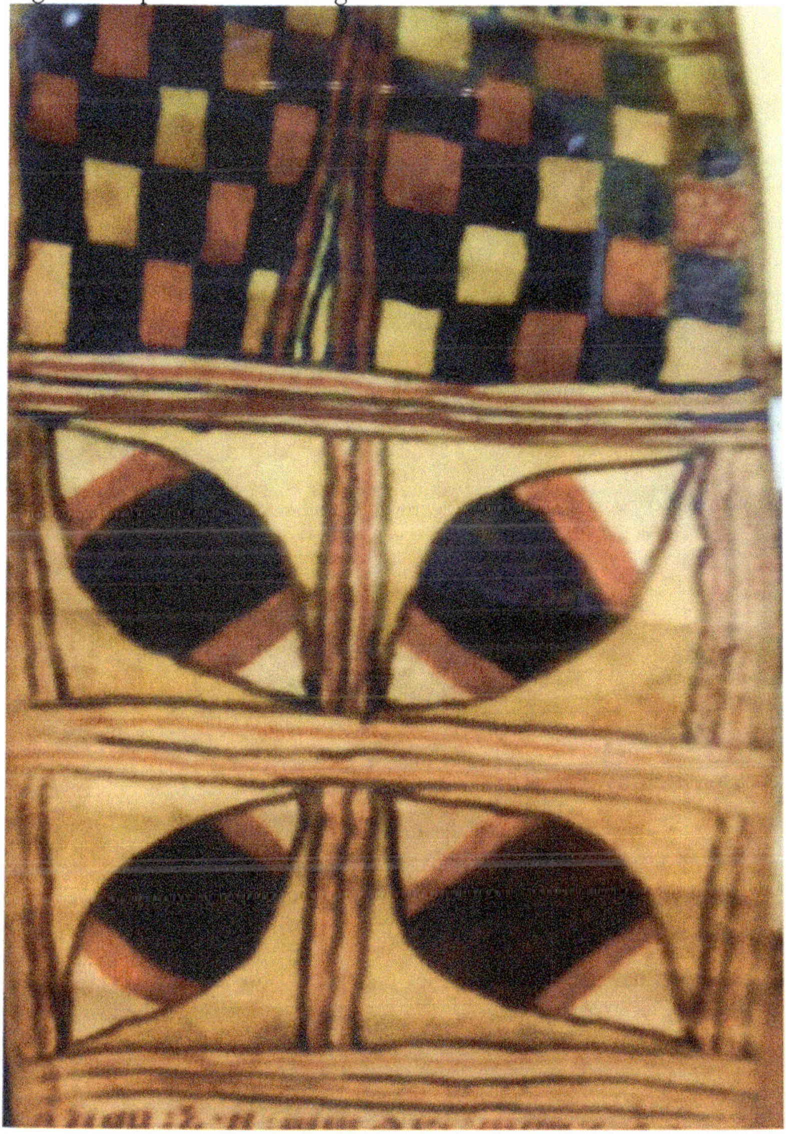

Source: Courtesy of IES

Figure 2: A magical drawing on a personal amulet

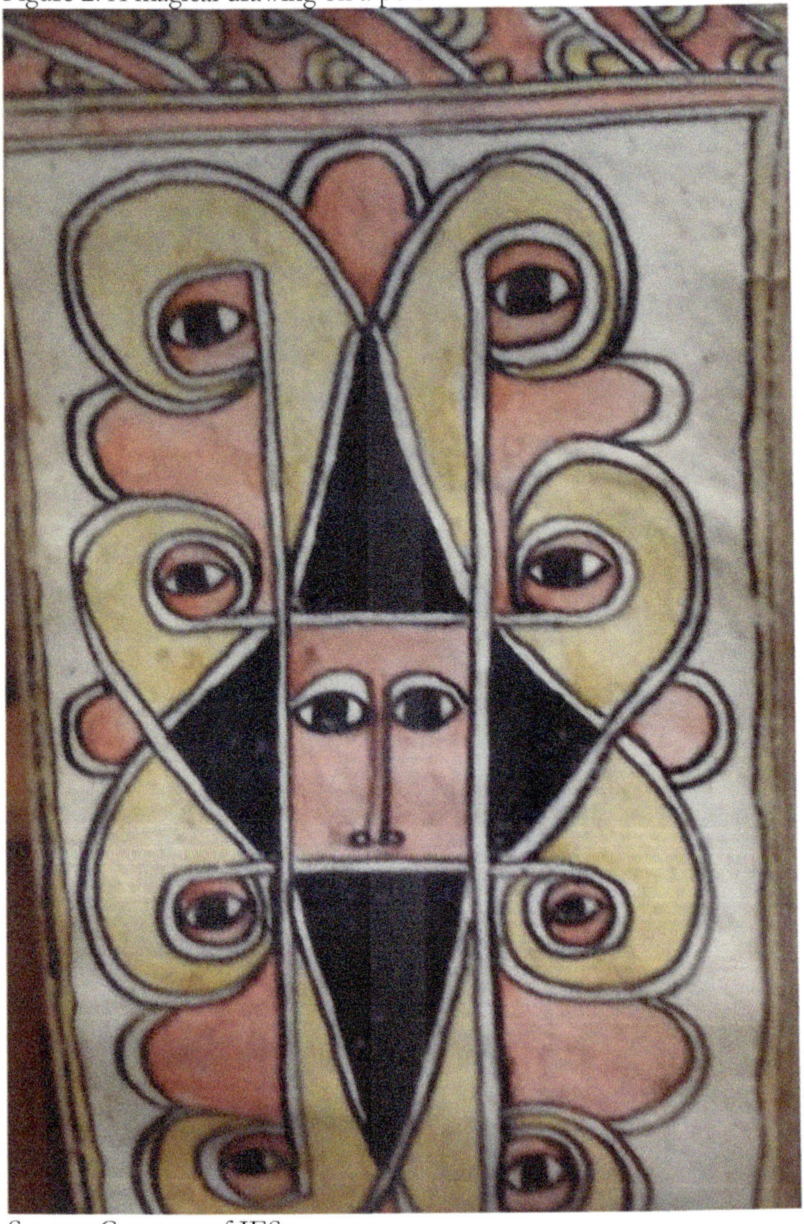

Source: Courtesy of IES

Notes

1 In Ethiopia about 11 500 traditional birth attendants were trained during the Darg regime, see Kebede Deribe et al., 'A Historical Overview of Traditional Medicine Practices and Policy in Ethiopia', *Ethiopian Journal of Health Development* 20(2) (2006): p. 130.

2 Mekonnen Bishaw, 'Promoting Traditional Medicine in Ethiopia: Brief Historical Review of Government Policy', *Social Science and Medicine* 33(2) (1991): p. 197.

3 Ibid., p. 199.

4 Stacy Pigg. 'Acronyms and Effacement: Traditional Medical Practitioners (TMPs) in International Health Development', *Social Science and Medicine* 41 (1995): pp. 59–60.

5 Edward Green and Lydia Makhubu, 'Traditional Healers in Swaziland: Toward Improved Cooperation between the Traditional and Modern Health Sectors', *Social Science and Medicine*, 18(12) (1984): p. 1077.

6 World Health Organization, *Primary Health Care: Report of the International Conference on Primary Health Care*, Alma-Ata, USSR, 6 to 12 September 1978 (Geneva: WHO, 1978).

7 Sjaak van der Geest, 'Is There a Role for Traditional Medicine in Basic Health Service in Africa? A Plea for a Community Perspective,' *Tropical Medicine and International Health* 2(9) (1997): p. 903. Geest has been very sceptical about the possibility of integration and tended to advocate the expansion of modern health infrastructure.

8 Stacy Pigg, 'Acronyms and Effacement', p. 64.

9 Ibid., p. 64.

10 Chunhuei Chi, 'Integrating Traditional Medicine into Modern Health Care Systems: Examining the Role of Chinese Medicine in Taiwan', *Social Science and Medicine* 39(3) (1994): p. 316

11 Scholars have identified four models of integration, namely (1) exclusive or monopolistic, (2) tolerant, (3) inclusive and (4) integrated.

12 Komila Tsey, 'Traditional Medicine in Contemporary Ghana: A Public Policy Analysis', *Social Science and Medicine* 45(7) (1997): 1065-1074.

13 Daniel Offiong, 'Traditional Healers in the Nigerian Health Care Delivery System and the Debate over Integrating Traditional and Scientific', *Anthropological Quarterly* 72(3) (1999): p. 118.

14 Geest, 'Is There a Role for Traditional Medicine?' p. 908; and also Velimirovic who has been highly critical of the 'integrationist' perspective saying that a 'genuine integration' has not taken place anywhere in the world. See Boris Velimirovi, 'Is Integration of Traditional and Western Medicine Really Possible?' in *Anthropology and*

Primary Health Care, edited by J. Coreil and J. D. Mull (Boulder, CO: West View Press, 1990), pp. 51-78.

15 John Janzen's *The Quest for Therapy in Lower Zaire* (Berkeley: University of California Press, 1979) remains a classic study of this pattern of health-seeking behaviour.

16 Randall M. Packard, *The Making of a Tropical Disease: A Short History of Malaria* (Baltimore: Johns Hopkins University Press, 2007), p. xii.

17 For a brief historical survey on state efforts to register and tax traditional healers since the colonial period, see Edward Green and Lydia Makhubu, 'Traditional Healers in Swaziland', *Social Science and Medicine* 18(12) (1984): 1071–1079. Formal training for traditional birth attendants was undertaken in at least 44 developing countries, including Ethiopia, but 'there are only one or two countries' that included traditional healers into their national health care systems'. For a comprehensive policy analysis and evaluation of the integration effort, see Barbara Pillsbury, 'Policy and Evaluation Perspectives on Traditional Health Practitioners in National Health Care Systems', *Social Science and Medicine* 16 (1982): pp. 1825–1834; A. K. Neumann and P. Lauro, 'Ethnomedicine and Biomedicine Linking', *Social Science and Medicine* 16 (1982): 1817–1824; Allan Young, 'The Relevance of Traditional Medical Culture to Modern Primary Health Care', *Social Science and Medicine* 17 (1983): pp. 1205–1211; Olayiwola Akerele, 'The Best of Both Worlds: Bringing Traditional Medicine up to Date', *Social Science and Medicine* 24(2) (1987): pp. 177–181; Leendert Slikkerveer, 'Rural Health Development in Ethiopia: Problems of Utilization of Traditional Healers', *Social Science and Medicine* 16 (1982): 1859–1872.

18 Mekonnen has highlighted the attitude of the successive Ethiopian governments towards indigenous medicine and the potential value of integrating indigenous healing into the biomedical system. See Mekonnen Bishaw. 'Integrating Indigenous and Cosmopolitan Medicine in Ethiopia', unpublished PhD dissertation (Southern Illinois University, 1988).

19 Amhara constituted what are today north Shewa, north and south Gondar, east and west Gojjam, and north and south Wallo. The capital of the State of Amhara, founded in 1996, is Bahir-Dar. The Amhara state shares common borders with the regional states of Tigray in the north, Afar in the east, Oromiya in the south, Benishangul/Gumuz in the southwest, and the Republic of Sudan in the west. It covers an estimated area of 170 752 square kilometres. According to the first official census of 1994, the region's population was 13 834 297 of which 90% was rural. Based on the same census, 81.5% of the population was Orthodox Christian. Regarding ethnic composition,

91.2% is Amhara, about 3% Oromo, 3.7% Agaw and 1.2% Qimant. See http://www.ethiopar.net/English/basinfo/infoamra.htm.

20 The informants fall into seven age groups: (1) 3 (4.7%) in their early eighties; (2) 4 (6.4%) in their late seventies; (3) 18 (28.6%) between their late sixties and early seventies; (4) 14 (22.2%) in their early sixties; (5) 13 (20.6%) in their late fifties; (6) 7 (11.1%) in their early fifties and the remaining (7) 4 (6.4%) are in their early forties.

21 Marcel Griaule, *Le livre de recettes d'un dabtara abyssin* (Paris: L'institut d'ethnologie, 1930); Deborah Lifchitz, *Textes ethioipiens magico-religieux* (Paris: L'institut d'ethnologie, 1940); Stefan Strelcyn, 'La magie Ethiopienne' (Rome: Academia Nazionale dei Lincei, 1960); Maxim Rodinson, *Magie, medicine possession en Ethiopie* (Paris: Mouton & Co., 1967).

22 For example, the French ethnologist Deborah Lifchitz analysed material that became important for the study of the magico-religious literature in Ethiopia. Sylvain Grebaut, who published innumerable Ge'ez texts in the journal, *Aethiopica*, was more concerned about the study of Ge'ez literature. The peculiarity of magic scrolls seems to have fascinated Grebaut into publishing a number of written amulets or magico-medical prayers in the journal of which he was the chief editor. (See, for instance, Michel Leiris, 'Le culte des Zars a Gondar', *Aethiopica* (1934); Michel Leiris, 'Un rite medico-magique ethiopien: Le jet de Danqara', *Aethiopica* (1934), and Michel Leiris, *La croyance aux genies "Zar" en Ethiopie du Nord.* (Paris, Librairie Felix Alcan, 1938), Grebaut, Sylvain, 'Priere magique contre la dysenterie,' *Aethiopica* (1934); Grebaut, Sylvain, 'Priere contre la pleuresie,' *Aethiopica* (1936); Grebaut, Sylvain, 'Priere magique contre le feu,' *Aethiopica*, (1936); Grebaut, Sylvain, 'Priere magique contre la grele,' *Aethiopica* (1938); Sebastien Euringer, 'l'hymne-invocation lessane sab'e', *Aethiopica* (1935); Grebaut, Sylvain, 'La priere sayfa malakot', *Aethiopica* (1936). People such as Grebaut were the ones who encouraged the study of magico-medical texts in Ethiopian studies. Some of them also collected a sizeable number of Ethiopian manuscripts in Europe. The texts are particularly important to identify medicinal plants and their scientific or Latin botanical names. In this regard, the exhaustive works of Strelcyn have no parallel: Stefan Strelcyn, *Medicins et plantes d'Ethiopie: Les traites medicaux ethiopiens*, volume 1. (Warazawa: Panstwowe, 1968); Stefan Strelcyn, *Medecine et plantes d'Ethiopie*, volume 2 (Naples: Instituto Universario Orientale, 1973).

23 Francisco Alvarez, *The Prester John of the Indies*, 2 volumes, revised and edited by C. F. Beckingham and G.W.B. Huntingford (Cambridge: Cambridge University Press, 1961). This sixteenth-century observation

was followed by Almeida's seventeenth-century and Bruce's eighteenth-century accounts. See Manoel de Almeida, *Some Records of Ethiopia, 1593–1646*, revised and edited by C. F. Beckingham and G.W.B. Huntingford (London: Hakluyt Society, 1954); James Bruce, *Travels to Discover the Source of the Nile in the Years 1768, 1769, 1770 1771, 1772, and 1773*, 5 volumes (London: G. G. J. and J. Robinson, 1970).

24 Allan Young, 'Medical Beliefs and Practices of Begemder Amhara', unpublished PhD dissertation (University of Pennsylvania, 1970).

25 Allan Young, 'Magic as a Quasi-Profession: The Organization of Magic and Magical Healing Among the Amhara.' *Ethnology* 14(3) (1975): pp. 245-265.

26 Allan Young, 'The Practical Logic of Amhara Traditional Medicine', in *African Therapeutic Systems*, edited by Z.A. Ademuwagun, et al (Massachusetts: Crossroads Press, 1979), pp. 132-137.

27 See Allan Young, 'Order, Analogy and Efficacy in Ethiopian Medical Divination,' *Culture, Medicine and Psychiatry* 1(2) 1977: pp. 183-199.

28 Simon Messing, 'The Highland Plateau Amhara of Ethiopia', unpublished PhD dissertation (University of Pennsylvania, 1957).

29 Mekonnen Bishaw, 'Integrating Indigenous and Cosmopolitan Medicine in Ethiopia', unpublished PhD dissertation (Southern Illinois University, 1988).

30 Dan Bauer, 'The Sacred and the Secret: Order and Chaos in Tigray Medicine and Politics', in *Creativity of Power*, edited by W. Arens and Ivan Karp (Washington, DC: Smithsonian Institution Press, 1989), pp. 225–243; Dan Bauer and John Hinnant, 'Normal and Revolutionary Divination: A Kuhnian Approach to African Systems of Thought', in *Explorations of African Systems of Thought* edited by Ivan Karp and Charles Bird, (Bloomington: Indiana University Press, 1979), pp. 213–236.

31 His other works included the history of cholera, typhus, smallpox, rabies, syphilis, influenza, leprosy and skin diseases. His book *An Introduction to the Medical History of Ethiopia* (Trenton: The Red Sea Press, 1990) is largely a collection of his previous works. See, for example, Richard Pankhurst, 'The History and Traditional Treatment of Small-pox in Ethiopia', *Medical History* 9(4) (1965); Richard Pankhurst, 'Traditional Ethiopian Medicine and Surgery', *Ethiopian Medical Journal* 3 (1965); Richard Pankhurst, 'Old-time Ethiopian Cures for Syphilis', *Journal of the History of Medicine and Allied Sciences* 30(3) (1975).

32 Richard Pankhurst, *An Introduction to The Medical History of Ethiopia* (Trenton: The Red Sea Press, 1990).

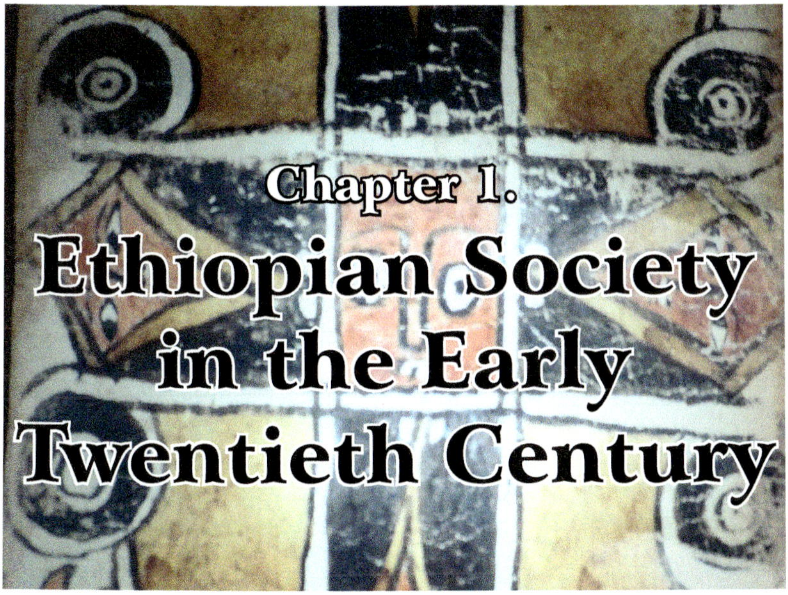

Chapter 1. Ethiopian Society in the Early Twentieth Century

To fully understand the history of church-based healing in Ethiopia during the twentieth century and its relationship to the state, it must be placed within the wider history of dramatic social, political and economic changes that have marked this period, for in a variety of ways these broader changes have shaped the development of healing practices and the status of church-based healing over the course of most of the twentieth century. This chapter begins by briefly examining early efforts on the part of successive Ethiopian rulers to so-called modernise, or Westernise, parts of Ethiopian society, including health care, from the middle of the nineteenth century through the early decades of the twentieth century. It also explains how these efforts shaped the medical landscape of Ethiopia at the beginning of the twentieth century.

Modernising Ethiopia

The Ethiopian highlands, which is the focus of this book and forms the centre of the current Ethiopian state, was the site of an ancient Ethiopian empire dating back to the fourth century CE. At the start of the nineteenth century, however, the region was fractured politically among a number of feudal princes struggling to gain dominance over it. The throne of the ancient Ethiopian empire, at Gondar, was occupied by the appointee of whichever prince or warlord succeeded in gaining control of the capital. Regions such as Gojjam and Shewa were ruled by their own branches of the imperial dynasty, and in Shewa the local prince went as far as assuming the title of king. The ethnically diverse population of the region generally adhered to the Orthodox Christian faith, which had been introduced into Ethiopia in the fourth century. However, successive Muslim incursions had occurred since the sixteenth century and during the nineteenth century the highlands were threatened by Muslim invasions from the north.[1]

In 1855 an ambitious local rebel seized control of Gondar and established himself as emperor, assuming the name Tewordos II. This event began a period of reunification and reform which, by the beginning of the twentieth century, had resulted in the re-establishment of a strong centralised Ethiopian state. Tewordos sought to unify and modernise Ethiopia, and within a short period after ascending the throne he was able to establish his authority over the warlords of Wallo and Tigray, and forcibly reincorporate the regions of Gojjam, Shewa and Wallo under the direct administration of the imperial throne. In addition, Tewordos sought to solidify his control by seeking help from a fellow Christian ruler, Queen Victoria of Britain. Tewordos asked that skilled craftspeople, knowledgeable in the manufacturing of firearms and other technologies, be sent to Ethiopia to help modernise his kingdom and defend it against Muslim incursions. The letter never reached the queen and it did not produce the desired results. Instead, it led to a major misunderstanding which eventually caused the British to dispatch a punitive expedition to Ethiopia in 1868. The expedition defeated the Ethiopian army and led Tewordos to kill himself.[2]

Tewordos was succeeded by a rival who had helped the British defeat Tewordos's army and in return received a large supply of firearms, which he employed to establish himself as Emperor Yohannes IV in 1872. Yohannes succeeded in maintaining the unity of the state that Tewordos had established, but he was forced to devote most of his energies to defending his empire from a series of invaders from the north, beginning with Khedive Isma'il Pasha of

Egypt, who sought to bring the entire Nile River Basin under his rule, and ending with the Muslim armies of the Madhist Revolt in the Sudan. Yohannes's preoccupation with the north forced him to allow the growth of Shewa autonomy to the south under the leadership of Menelik. Menelik took advantage of his autonomy and Shewa's trade wealth to expand his kingdom to the south and east. When Yohannes was killed in battle with the Mahdist forces, Menelik was in a position to claim the imperial throne.[3]

Menelik followed the efforts begun by Tewordos II to modernise Ethiopia. Like Tewordos, he sought to align himself with a European power, signing a treaty recognising Italian control over parts of northern Tigray, which became the colony of Eritrea. The Italians, however, claimed that the treaty gave them control over the whole of Ethiopia, leading Menelik to reject the treaty. The Italians responded to this rejection by invading Ethiopia from Eritrea. Menelik, whose military forces were well armed, succeeded in defeating the Italians at the battle of Adwa, preserving his country's independence.[4]

However, the Battle of Adwa forced Menelik to reassess his situation. While he had succeeded in temporarily halting the European advance, his country was surrounded by a ring of European colonies, namely the British in the Sudan, Kenya and Somalia; the Italians in Eritrea and Somalia; and the French in Djibouti. In addition, the Europeans, in defiance of Ethiopia's claims to sovereignty, were constructing treaties among themselves that threatened Ethiopia's political and economic interests.[5]

Associating his country's vulnerability with its technological backwardness, Menelik shifted his attention to Westernising his realm.[6] Soon the imperial capital at Addis Ababa 'became crowded with foreign embassies determined to negotiate treaties, demarcate borders, establish commercial relations, and gain concessions. Merchants, agents, adventurers, and freebooters of all types also descended on [the capital] . . . seeking contracts, franchises, orders, or jobs as advisers, interpreters, craftsmen, mercenaries, etc.'[7]

Menelik's contacts with foreign nationals provided him with the opportunity to learn about European technological innovations and economic progress. Building on this knowledge, he began constructing hospitals, pharmacies, a public school, a municipality, a police force and a ministerial system of government.[8] He also continued to modernise his army, and extend the railway and telegraph services.

Menelik's modernisation efforts, however, did not transform the country's economy, which remained largely feudal and was based on the appropriation of large tracts of agricultural lands either as *rist* (hereditary landownership), *gult* (non-hereditary system of landownership) or *rista gult* (*gult* lands changed hereditarily). The emperor was, in theory and to a considerable degree in practice, the owner of all land in the empire, and those who worked on the land were literally tenants of the emperor. The labour of these tenants supported the government, the landowning class and the church.[9]

The Ethiopian Orthodox Tewahedo Church, related to the Egyptian Coptic Orthodox Church, was a powerful force in Ethiopia. It claimed the adherence of much of the country's highland population, bolstered the political authority of the emperor, who was its titular head, and had tremendous economic power based on its possession of vast tracts of agricultural lands cultivated either by the clergy themselves or by peasants of the neighbouring villages.[10]

Slave raiding was also an important source of wealth to most members of the upper nobility.[11] The institutions of slavery and slave trade had been maintained for a long time, and were not abolished until the early 1920s, at which point an imperial decree was issued to eliminate these practices in a gradual manner. The final abolition of these practices, which was made possible through external and internal pressures, was indeed a gradual process.[12]

Menelik's Westernising efforts faced resistance from various quarters.[13] Opposition was particularly visible in the area of Western education, which the Orthodox clergy and their adherents viewed as a challenge to their faith and the integrity of the traditional educational system. Religious leaders were at the forefront of resistance against new ideas, for they had little trouble mobilising the laity in the name of defending their age-old traditions and faith. Believing that new ideas would corrupt the young and the established system, some groups viewed the importation and 'idolisation' of Western ideas as both strange and impious. They even doubted the soundness of the emperor's mental condition.[14]

It was not easy for Menelik to move fast with his Westernisation plan. Each move met with resistance; for example, he tried to introduce a mechanical grinding machine to replace the traditional one. Menelik viewed hand grinding as labour-intensive, unhygienic and subject to contamination. However, the clergy viewed the new mechanical grinder as the work of the devil and, along with the nobility, preferred to have teff grain *injera* (a yeast-risen flatbread) powdered with a hand-mill.[15] Menelik's challenge in helping acquaint his entourage with footwear was no less serious than to efforts to introduce the grinding machine. Those who wore shoes were stigmatised as 'lepers' or as lacking a sturdy foot, a symbol of unmanly behaviour; even Menelik's grandson lacked the courage to embrace his ideas.[16]

Attempts to introduce Western education were of particular concern to church leaders, because for several centuries the country's educational system had been the responsibility of churches and monasteries.[17] These religious institutions produced a limited number of literate individuals—scribes or *dabtara*, some priests[18] and a handful of high-ranking individuals—who could read and write.[19] Dr Mérab, a Georgian physician working in Ethiopia for many decades, noted in the early twentieth century that only 10 per cent among the Amhara population as a whole and about 1 in 1 000 among the womenfolk were literate.[20] In the early 1930s Griaule estimated that there were only a few literate priests numbering 'about one in ten of the population' of Gojjam.[21] It was, in part, the limited extent to which the church had succeeded in producing a literate population that led Menelik to turn to Western education. He brought 15 teachers from Coptic Egypt,[22] the patriarchate that supplied bishops to the Ethiopian church up to the 1950s. These Egyptian teachers began to work in the first public school that the emperor had founded in Addis Ababa in 1908.[23] Yet the resistance of the Orthodox Church persisted and Western education made little headway.

The Introduction of Western Medicine

By comparison, Menelik's effort to popularise foreign medicines and medical treatments seemed less challenging. He was relatively successful in persuading the nobility to take advantage of the available biomedical products. As Pankhurst pointed out, Western medicine 'made headway at first in royal and princely circles, and later

[it] gained currency among the nobility, and more generally, among the population of capitals and other centers of political power'.[24] This state of affairs confirmed the 'top–bottom' approach to foreign medicine in Ethiopia.

Yet for most of Menelik's subjects at the beginning of the twentieth century, nearly all human misfortunes were attributed to the machinations of evil-intended persons and a host of disease-causing spiritual beings. Menelik's incapacitating illness, presumably high blood pressure, was variously ascribed to a magic spell cast by the proverbial black cat, criminal poisoning, an envious gaze of the evil eye and even to the influence of a 'devil-fabricated automobile in which he rode for the first time.[25] These outlooks, reflecting the mindset of the time, had strong currency among the clergy who exerted tremendous pressure on the emperor to terminate the biomedical care he was receiving from foreign physicians and to continue with his treatment of holy water.[26] Reflecting on the indigenous cosmological beliefs of the early twentieth century, Gebre Hiywot wrote that no one in the world sought the assistance of good and bad spirits more than Ethiopian rulers.[27]

To ease public anxiety caused by his newly introduced ideas, Menelik sought a suitable compromise between the indigenous and Western therapeutic systems. As part of this scheme, he provided experienced healers with full-time employment at Arada Clinic, a branch of the Menelik Hospital,[28] which was staffed almost entirely by salaried church-educated healers.[29] One of the clerics, Gabrawald, a physician and a specialist in leprosy, haemorrhoids, scrofula and syphilis, received a yearly salary of 30 Maria Theresa dollars, along with butter and honey; and he continued his service during the Haile Selassie era.[30] However, the official encouragement provided to indigenous healers was entirely confined to the imperial capital and had no impact on the majority of healers working in the rest of the country.[31]

Although appreciative of the virtues of foreign medicine, Menelik seemed to encourage allopathic medicine only as long as it maintained a compromising stance towards indigenous therapeutics. To create a 'curious compromise between traditional and western medicine', the Russian Medical Mission that came to Ethiopia following the battle of Adwa was asked by Emperor Menelik to produce the 'first western Amharic [bio]medical textbook [or manual]'.[32]

Despite his interest in Western biomedicine, Menelik did not refrain from tapping the expertise of indigenous healers. In 1901 he wrote a letter asking Alaqa Gefawossen, a renowned cleric–healer, to travel to Yejju (Wallo) to treat Ras (a title, roughly equivalent to Duke or Lord) Wolle, his brother-in-law.[33] Indigenous medical knowledge was a valuable resource that served the needs of members of the royal court and state officials.[34] The emperor himself sought out both Western and indigenous healers to help with his distressing illness. Recognising the services of indigenous health practitioners, Menelik II rewarded a distinguished cleric–healer by the name of Qese Gebez Iskezziah Wolde. Iskezziah was so famous for his service that 'even foreigners came to see him'.[35] Observing the use of European medicine by the Ethiopian political leaders, Merid wrote: 'Yohannes IV, Menelik II, Taitu, Zawditu, Iyasu, Haile Selassie and their ministers were well under the thumbs of their European doctors.'[36]

Likewise, the public, although highly sceptical of the therapeutic modalities of newly introduced biomedical treatments, did not wholly resist the services of the new health facilities.[37] This receptive tendency was developed through contacts with European travellers and residents who had come to Ethiopia with 'chests full of tablets, powders and ointments' since the second half of the nineteenth century. These non-professional foreign nationals may be regarded as the pioneers of European healing methods in the country.[38]

Pankhurst has spotlighted the availability 'to the richer classes or those with access to imported drugs [such as sarsaparilla and calomel or chloride of mercury]' of new forms of treatments against syphilis.[39] The treatment against venereal diseases was one of 'the medical field[s] in which the Ethiopian public was perhaps most responsive to change'.[40] Provision of treatments against syphilis and Jenner-type vaccines against smallpox were important areas of competition among European legations working tirelessly to open up the country for Western medicine.[41]

The Russian Red Cross Mission established the first hospital in Addis Ababa in 1897. It offered free medical services to the inhabitants of the capital.[42] This free service was not warmly received due partly to the strong *vis inertiae* of the church which made the public highly mistrustful of the *ferengi* (whites) and their medicine.[43] In

1907 a unit called *Bureau de l'Hygiene Publique* was set up in the Ministry of the Interior, one of Menelik's ministerial offices. A year later the first government hospital, the Menelik Hospital, was established and the first pharmacy, Pharmacia L'Georgia, owned by Dr Mérab, was opened in Addis Ababa in 1910. The limited biomedical products put up for sale in the pharmacies were expensive and were sold alongside indigenous Ethiopian medicines, 'among these was the taenicide *kosso*' (variously known as *Hagenia abyssinica*).[44]

The sale of imported and indigenous remedies in the pharmacies clearly indicates the public's receptivity to the incursions of Western drugs, particularly if they did not render the underlying principles of Ethiopian medicine obsolete. However, the limited variety of drugs available prevented allopathic medicine from establishing its authority over other forms of healing; for example, the drugs and treatments of biomedicine proved ineffective to cope with the pandemic influenza or Spanish 'flu' of 1918, known locally as 'Yahedar Basheta' (November's Disease).[45] Realising the futility of biomedicine, the urban public resorted to the indigenous preventative and/or therapeutic schemes: these included retreating to remote or disease-free areas and seeking out remedies from indigenous healers. Recourse to the traditional medicaments such as the leaves of eucalyptus (*Bahr zaf*), local alcoholic drinks and *nech shenkurt* (*Allium cepa*), either as prophylactic or therapeutic items, was widely reported.[46]

Western medicine recognised the difficulty of getting a strong foothold in a medical landscape dominated by a variety of indigenous practitioners: church-based healers (*dabtara*), so named because they began their education as ecclesiastical students in church schools, and possessed the widest array of medical knowledge; herbalists; and secular and spiritual practitioners of various titles, such as bone-setters and traditional birth attendants. Before becoming a dominant healthcare system, Western medicine had to endure scores of challenges and work in a pluralistic medical framework. It had to pass through three ostensibly interrelated phases, namely (1) the period of encroachment on the terrain of indigenous medicine; (2) competition with the indigenous medical system and (3) its virtual domination of a sizeable portion of the medical marketplace. It was not until the mid-1940s that Western medicine, which by then had established scientific claims to its medical authority, became an established system of health care in Ethiopia. Before then, it represented but one of many options available to patients seeking medical cures. The most important of these among Orthodox Christian Ethiopians was church-based healing.

The Medical Landscape

Before examining the role of church-based healing in Ethiopia and the challenges that it increasingly faced over the course of the twentieth century, one needs to examine the wide variety of indigenous medical practitioners who occupied the country's medical landscape at the beginning of the twentieth century.

Herbalist–healers were the largest group of specialists occupying the early twentieth-century medical landscape. The art of herbal therapy was the oldest medical tradition in Ethiopia and, in all likelihood, it predated other forms of indigenous healing. Although all indigenous practitioners employed botanical medicine, it would be a mistake to designate all groups of healers as 'herbalists'. Here, the term 'herbalist' refers strictly to medical specialists who prepared and administered herbal drugs only. Though largely illiterate and dependent on memory to learn and preserve their medical information, the majority of herbalist–healers commanded an extensive knowledge of the plant kingdom. Acquiring herbal knowledge was a lengthy process, requiring prospective healers to undergo a long period of apprenticeship under the mentorship of experienced herbalists. The quality of medical training was crucial to produce proficient, God-fearing, ethically and morally abided herbalist–healers.[47]

The Zar-possessed or the *balazar* were the single most important group of spiritually inspired practitioners of the early twentieth century. The belief in the spirit of Zar, the former sky god of the Cushitic Agaw, had an ancient origin predating even the introduction of Christianity and Islam to Ethiopia. After Christianity had assumed spiritual predominance, however, the Zar was relegated to becoming a possessing spirit.[48] Scores of human maladies and tribulations were attributed to the Zar spirit in Ethiopia, as well as in neighbouring countries and areas of the Arabian peninsula.[49]

When an intrusion of a disease-causing spirit was suspected, a person with a history of Zar spirit possession was found right away to serve as a spirit medium and communicate with the spirit causing the sickness. During these ritual healing sessions, the Zar spirit, through its human medium, would identify the troubling spirit, including Jinn and evil eye spirits, diagnose the illness and recommend a therapeutic solution. Spiritually inspired healers, using their clairvoyant powers, recommended various kinds of therapeutic modalities to the physically ill, the psychologically disturbed, and to those with scores of personal and social problems.

Another group of secular practitioners was called the *waggesha* (lit. 'the one who gives relief' or 'the one who effects a cure').[50] The term *waggesha* or 'surgeon–herbologist–empricist[s]'[51] stood for indigenous healers who, in large part, effected cures through the physical manipulation of the human body. Like the majority of herbalist–healers, the *waggesha* were mostly non-literate and mustered no esoteric or mystic knowledge. They acquired their craft through a long period of apprenticeship. Written records on the *waggesha*'s empirico-therapeutic vocations date from the sixteenth century; they served as bone-setters (or orthopaedists) and performed other surgical operations, such as cauterisation, bleeding, cupping, circumcision, cutting the uvula, scarification, opening abscesses, removing tumours and bullets, and extracting carious teeth.[52] In addition to these specialised skills, the *waggesha* also possessed a limited amount of herbal knowledge; essentially pragmatic and experiential wisdom.

Paramount among the wide array of practitioners of indigenous medicine, church-based healers were viewed as particularly skilled in treating an exceptionally broad range of medical and social problems. Church-based healers who possessed the widest array of magico-medical knowledge had to undergo the most rigorous training, involving, as explained in the next chapter, years of education from a range of teachers located over wide areas of the country. It was only after this long period of textually based and practical training that medical students could command the religious, linguistic and magico-medical subjects needed to practise their craft. Though the history of church-based medical education can be traced back to the early days of the Orthodox Church, the earliest magico-medical manuscripts identified so far belonged to the seventeenth century.[53] Religious institutions played a decisive role in providing the instructional resources for church-based medicine and healing for several centuries, even though, as will become evident, the church viewed the acquisition of medical knowledge with some trepidation. The training of cleric–healers resulted in their acquisition of the wisdom to invoke and exorcise evil spirits; cast and break magic spells; make divinations; provide herbal treatments; and produce written amulets and talismans.

The availability of indigenous practitioners of differing educational background and training, as well as their competition for the medical market, was a major feature of the medical landscape of the early twentieth century. It is worth noting that the success of any group of healers within this market was determined not simply by the group's ability to attract patients, but also by the extent to which any given medical tradition was sanctioned by the political elites and the church. The role of the church and state in influencing the medical marketplace continued to be a dominant feature of the history of therapeutics over the course of the twentieth century.

The Medical Landscape after Menelik

The death of Menelik in 1913 occurred at the time when Western allopathic medicine was beginning to make steady incursions into the medical marketplace. Indigenous medical specialists, cognisant of the impending threat that Western medicine posed, adopted gestures to accommodate it and this helped them gain time to learn about its limitations.

The pressure of Western medicine on indigenous healers was limited in the immediate post-Menelik era; a period characterised by internal strife and power struggles. The Ethiopian government did not take an official stance on indigenous medicine. The 1934 government regulation that laid down the conditions under which biomedical practitioners should register and practise[54] did not talk about the status of indigenous health practitioners nor did it interdict or make illegal their medical activity. Indigenous healers had little difficulty exercising their 'occupational rights'.

Subsequent Ethiopian rulers, however, made efforts to expand biomedical institutions. Emperor Haile Selassie I (r. 1930–1974), alias 'Ras Tefari' before his coronation, was particularly notable in this respect.[55] Despite 'the disdainful attitude of the Ethiopians in general and the active opposition of the Church',[56] Haile Selassie supported missionary societies involved in the field of healthcare and education.[57]

Yet cosmopolitan medicine made little real progress before the Italian occupation of Ethiopia in the mid-1930s. In addition, the diffusion of biomedical institutions in the provinces was much slower than in the capital;[58] for instance, before the Italian invasion, a clinic attached to the Italian commercial agency and a hospital run by the American Seventh Day Adventist Mission rendered a limited amount of medical care to the people of Dessie town.[59] However, the people were not enthusiastic about exploiting the medical services of the missionaries. The Orthodox clergy misconstrued the missionaries as 'Catholics' or 'untrue Christians', and this prevented the laity from using these medical establishments.[60] The idea of religious contamination had a strong currency among the people of the Amhara region.

However, as access to Western medicine grew following the Italian invasion in 1935, indigenous healers of all types, especially church-based healers, found themselves having to cope with efforts to control their activities and subordinate them to Western medicine. At times, these efforts involved overt attacks on healers. It took a long time for indigenous healers to obtain the sympathy of the state and to be legally sanctioned as health practitioners. By the time this occurred, church-based medicine had undergone considerable change. To understand the nature of this change, adequate information on the practice of church-based medicine and education as it existed in the 1920s and 1930s is needed.

Figure 3: Preventive magical prayer against evils spirits

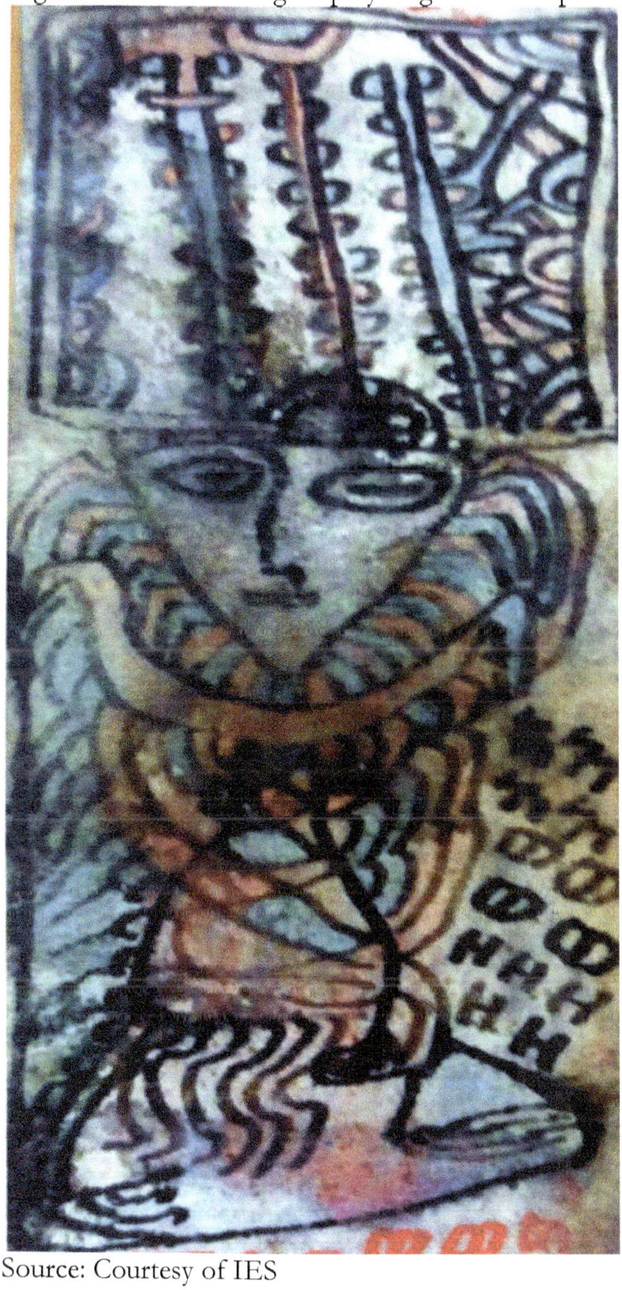

Source: Courtesy of IES

Figure 4: A written amulet to ward off disease-causing spirits

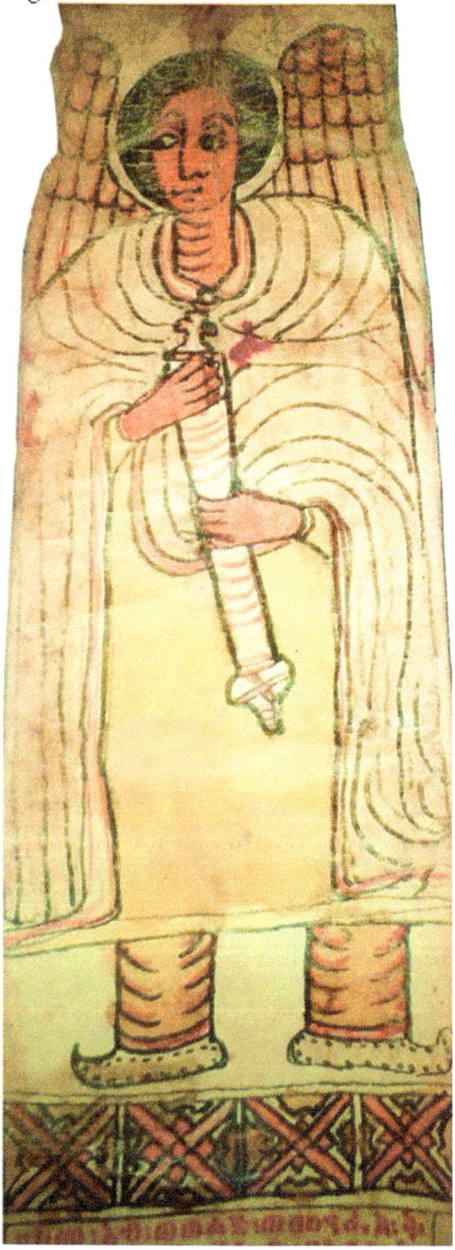

Source: IES Ms. No. 443

Figure 5: A personal amulet for keeping noxious spirits away

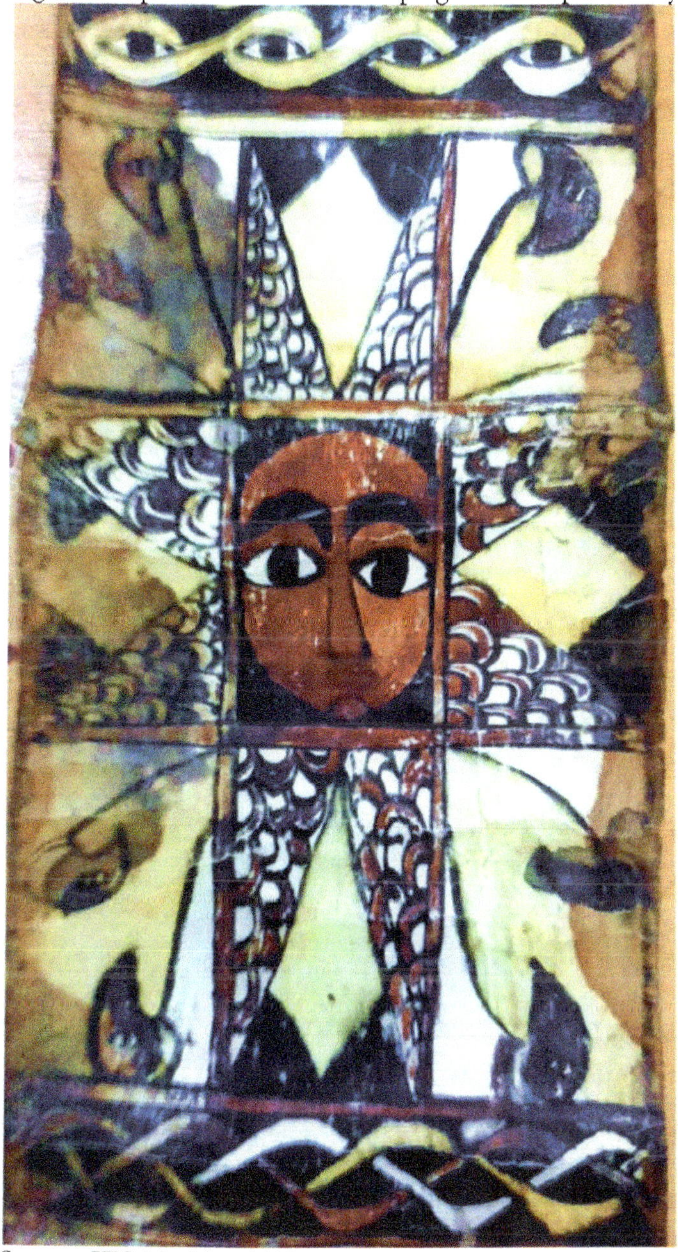

Source: IES Ms. No. 4448

Notes

1 Mordechai Abir, *Ethiopia and the Red Sea: The Rise and Decline of the Solomonic Dynasty and Muslim-European Rivalry in the Region* (London: Frank Cass and Company Limited, 1980), 69–101.

2 Harold G. Marcus, *A History of Ethiopia* (Berkeley: University of California Press, 1994), 70.

3 Richard Greenfield, *Ethiopia: A New Political History* (London: Pall Mall Press, 1965), 85–95.

4 Ibid, 115–118, 122–124.

5 The Tripartite Agreement between Britain, France and Italy in 1906, and that of the 1908 Franco-Ethiopian or the Klobukowsky Treaty were among such attempts to circumscribe Ethiopia's complete independence. As Bahru noted, Ethiopia 'found itself under the shadow of the same imperialism that was penetrating the colonial African economy', evolving into what may be termed a 'semi-colonial relationship' in which European capital began to have a foothold through concessions and trade. See Bahru Zewde, *A History of Modern Ethiopia, 1855–1974* (Addis Ababa: Addis Ababa University Press, 1991), 85.

6 Tekle Tsadik Mekuria, *Emperor Menelik and Ethiopian Unity* (Amharic) (Addis Ababa: Kuraz Publishing Agency, 1983 E.C.), 586.

7 John Markakis, *Ethiopia: Anatomy of a Traditional Polity* (Oxford: Clarendon Press, 1974), 144.

8 Pawlos Gnogno, *Atse Menelik* (Amharic) (Addis Ababa: Bole Printing Press, 1984 E.C.).

9 It was with the Proclamation no. 31/1975 that tenancy was abolished and peasants were freed from all obligations to landlords or the church.

10 Kristin Chaillot, *The Ethiopian Orthodox Tewahedo Church Traditions*: A Brief Introduction to Its Life and Spirituality (Amharic), trans. Dagnachew Kassahun (Addis Ababa: Mahbere Qedusan, 1999 E.C.), 32.

11 The struggle to control a web of trade routes and customs duties was a source of strength and incessant conflict among the ruling elites. Bahru Zewde, *A History of Modern Ethiopia,* 94.

12 Ibid., 93–94.

13 For a collective biography of early twentieth-century Ethiopian intellectuals and their far-reaching influences on the social and political transformations of the country, see Bahru Zewde, *Pioneers of Change in Ethiopia: Reformist Intellectuals of the Early Twentieth Century* (Addis Ababa: Addis Ababa University Press, 2002). One of the intellectuals of this period who criticised Menelik for being slow in his civilising endeavours believed that the emperor was liable to commit mistakes because he

lacked precise development programmes and relied on foreign advisers. See Takla Hawariyat Takla Mariam, *Autobiography* (Amharic) (Addis Ababa: Addis Ababa University Press, 1998 E.C.) 158–161.

14 Tekle Tsadik Mekuria, *Emperor Menelik and Ethiopia's Unity*, 598.

15 Pawlos Gnogno, *Atse Menelik*, 338.

16 Rumour had it that it was to conceal his deformed feet that the emperor would want to wear shoes; and to disprove this, the emperor on occasion walked in public barefooted or putting on sandal shoes (as he mostly did in the past). This was to show that he had healthy feet and to encourage others to do the same. Ibid., 339.

17 Ibid., 576.

18 Ibid., 586.

19 Ibid., 589. For a brief assessment of the literacy situation in northern Ethiopia in the late nineteenth century, see Mansfeld Parkyns, *Life in Abyssinia*, vol. I (New York: D. Appleton & Co., 1854) 139; Samuel Gobat, *Journal of the Three Years' Residence in Abyssinia* (London: Hatchard & Son, Seeley & Sons, 1834), 312–313; Theophilius Waldmeier, *Autobiography* (London: The Orphans Printing Press, 1925), 16.

20 With regard to higher officials, 'only half the Council of Ministers could read and write with ease, that three could do neither, and that two others knew no more than how to sign their names'. Paul Mérab, *Impressions d'Ethiopie 1921–1929*, vol. III (Paris: Editions Ernest Leroux, 1921–1929), 343–347.

21 Marcel Griaule, 'Le travail en Abyssinie', *Revue Internationale du Travail*, 23(2) (1931): 7.

22 He did not bring teachers from Catholic France or the so-called anti-Mary England whose presence can well be traced back to the nineteenth century; Tekle Tsadik Mekuria, *Emperor Menelik and Ethiopian Unity*, 587.

23 Students were encouraged to pursue their education with 'pocket money of three [Maria] thalers and [a regular] meal from the palace'. Bahru Zewde, *Pioneers of Change*, 24.

24 Richard Pankhurst, *A Social History of Ethiopia* (Addis Ababa: Institute of Ethiopian Studies, 1990), 306.

25 Gebre Selassie (Tsehafi Tezaz), *A History of the Period of Menelik II, Emperor of Ethiopia* (Amharic) (Addis Ababa: Artistic Printing Press, 1959 E.C.), 339.

26 Pawlos Gnogno, *Atse Menelik*, 459.

27 Gebre Hiywot Baykedagne, *Emperor Menelik and Ethiopia*, 5.

28 Tsehai Berhane Selassie, 'An Ethiopian Medical Text-book Written by Gerazmac Gabrawald Aragahan Daga Damot', *JES*, 3(1) (1971): 98.

29 A cleric–healer who had been assigned as an 'internist' obtained the approval and certification from Dr Hamer, an expatriate physician

working in Addis Ababa. The other five healers, three of whom were *alaqa* (a church title, which literally means 'master' or 'teacher') also assumed various positions in the same clinic: director, administrator, secretary, oculist and surgeon, Tsehai Berhane Selassie, 'An Ethiopian Medical Text-book'; the person assigned as a surgeon must have been a talented *waggesha* (lit. 'bone-setter' or 'orthopaedist'). 98.

30 Ibid., 98.

31 Apart from Menelik's early twentieth-century efforts, his successor did not overly concern himself with the issue of integration.

32 The 22-page manual incorporated few indigenous medical practices. Richard Pankhurst, *An Introduction to the Medical History of Ethiopia* (Trenton: The Red Sea Press, 1990), 126.

33 ይድረስ ካለቃ ግፋ ወሰን እንዴት ሰንብተሃል እኔ እግዚአብሔር ይመስገን ደህና ነኝ ራስ ወሌ ታመዋልና ይህ ደብዳቤ እንደደረሰህ ተነስተህ ይህንን ደብዳቤ ይዞ ከመጣው ጋራ ሌት ከቀን ገስግሰህ የጁ ራስ ወሌ ድረስ እንድትሄድ ይሁን 'May this letter reach Alaqa Gefawossen. How have you been? Thanks to God, I am fine. Ras Wolle is sick. As soon as this letter reaches you, start traveling to Yejju to Ras Wolle day and night with the man who brings you this letter.' See the National Healers' Association, 'A Letter of Emperor Menelik to Alaqa Gefawossen', *Genbot* 13 (1893 E.C., 20 May 1901).

34 It was for the purpose of gathering information from prophet– or cleric–diviners and soothsayers that the imperial court was said to have appointed a *liqa matane* (literally 'an expert evaluator of legal matters', a title most probably replaced later with *afe negus* or 'mouthpiece of the king'), a person entrusted to evaluate and report the likely important divinatory information to the sovereign. See Tilahun Berhane Selassie, *Twentieth Century Ethiopia*, vol. 1 (Amharic) (Addis Ababa: Artistic Printing Press, 1998, E.C.), 400–401.

35 Reidulf Molvaer, 'Medical Anthropology Topics of Relevance for Health Workers and Students of Health in Ethiopia', (Addis Ababa: UNICEF/Ministry of Health, 1987), 25. Menelik seemed to have recognized Iskezziah's service as medical personnel during his numerous military campaigns.

36 Merid Wolde Aregay, 'Traditional Medical Practices in a Historical Perspective', paper read at the Annual Dinner of the Ethiopian Medical Association, *Mimeograph* (Addis Ababa, n.d (1987)), 9.

37 As Hasib Ydlibi, a concessionaire of the early twentieth century, wrote: 'All Abyssinians are . . . highly distrustful of European doctors . . . Even Menelik was no exception to this rule.' See May Ydlibi, *With Ethiopian Rulers: A Biography of Hasib Ydlibi*, edited by Bahru Zewde (Addis Ababa: Addis Ababa University Press, 2006), 134.

38 The 'medical' activity of these foreign nationals enabled the ruling elites and their families to profit from the rudiments, or what Charles Rosenberg would like to call the 'not-fully matured' allopathic medicine. See Charles Rosenberg, 'Alternative to What? Complementary to Whom?' paper presented to the Program in the History of Science, Medicine and Technology, The Johns Hopkins University, 14 September 2006.

39 Richard Pankhurst, 'Old-time Ethiopian Cures for Syphilis', *Journal of the History of Medicine and Allied Sciences*, 30(3) (1975): 216.

40 Richard Pankhurst, *A Social History of Ethiopia*, 309.

41 Richard Pankhurst, 'The Beginnings of Modern Medicine in Ethiopia', *Ethiopian Observer* volume 9(2) (1965): 131. Although his efforts did not bear much fruit, Menelik II went to the extent of outlawing the age-old inoculation methods against small pox. See Richard Pankhurst, 'The History and Traditional Treatment of Small-pox in Ethiopia', *Medical History* 9(4) (1965), 350–352.

42 Richard Pankhurst, 'The Beginnings of Modern Medicine', 129.

43 It must have been reminiscent of this strategy that the Ethiopian government in subsequent decades offered an almost free and highly subsidized medical service to the public.

44 Helmut Kloos and Others, 'The Geography of Pharmacies, Druggist Shops, and Rural Medicine Vendors, and the Origin of Customers to such Facilities in Addis Ababa', *JES*, 12(2) (1974): 81.

45 This global pandemic, according to Pankhurst, was the 'last major epidemic to hit the country before [sic] the advent of modern medical facilities'. For a detailed account of this devastating epidemic, see Richard Pankhurst, 'The *Hedar Bašeta* of 1918', *JES*, 13(2) (1975): 103–131. In contrast, the pandemic seemed to have advanced the cause of Western medicine in Ethiopia.

46 For a brief remark on the medicinal use and relative efficacy of *Bahr zaf* during this epidemic, see Imru Haile Selassie, *From What I Heard and Remember* (Amharic) (Addis Ababa: Addis Ababa University Press, 2001, E.C.), 89.

47 Most herbalists did not even accept payments from patients; and those who wanted to be remunerated demanded only nominal fees; a belief attributed to safeguarding the claimed potency of drug plants.

48 Spencer Trimingham, *Islam in Ethiopia* (London: Frank Cass & Co. Ltd. 1965), 27.

49 See Richard Natvig, 'Oromos, Slaves, and the Zar Spirits: A Contribution to the History of the Zar Cult,' *The International Journal of African Historical Studies*, 20(4) (1987): 647–668. There is extensive literature on the Zar cult; and the earliest written texts belonged to the

sixteenth century. More importantly, the early twentieth-century works of Marcel Griaule and Michel Leiris had definitely opened up the venue for more scholarly studies and interpretations of the Zar cult in Ethiopia. For ethnographic and analytical review of the literature on the Zar cult, see Harald Aspen, *Mediums and Human Worlds: The Amhara Peasants of the North Ethiopian Highlands and Their Traditions of Knowledge*, unpublished PhD dissertation (University of Trondhein, 1994), 45–64.

50 The word *waggesha* is an Oromo derivative which indicated the cultural influence of the Oromo people in the medical field.

51 Simon Messing, 'The Highland Plateau Amhara of Ethiopia', unpublished PhD dissertation (University of Pennsylvania, 1957), 580.

52 Richard Pankhurst, 'Historical Examination on the Traditional Ethiopian Pharmacopoeia,' paper presented at the Conference of the Ethiopian Pharmaceutical Association, 1975.

53 Ibid.

54 F.O., 371, no. 18028; 'The Ethiopian Order-in-Council', no. 2 of 1934.

55 When Tafari became regent in 1916, Addis Ababa had one governmental hospital and a public school, along with a few private and missionary medical and educational institutions. The extensive tours that he made to the outside world in 1924 persuaded the future emperor to become an avid admirer of European technological advancements. Richard Pankhurst, 'The Foundations of Education, Printing, Newspaper, Book Production, Libraries and Literacy in Ethiopia', *Ethiopian Observer*, 6(3) (1962): 266.

56 John Markakis, *Ethiopia: Anatomy of a Traditional Polity*, 146.

57 See Donald Crummey, 'The Politics of Westernization: Protestant and Catholic Missionaries in Western Ethiopia', in *The Missionary Factor in Ethiopia*, edited by Getatchew Haile et al. (Frankfurt am Main: 1998), 85ff.

58 During the Italian invasion there were about 18 hospitals in the country as a whole, 2 of which (the Menelik Hospital in Addis and the one in Gore) were governmental, while the other 16 were non-governmental and missionary hospitals serving in and outside Addis Ababa. See Mahatma Selassie Wolde Meskel, *Zekra Nagar: Recollection of Things Past* (Amharic), 2nd edition (Addis Ababa: Artistic Printing Press, 1962, E.C.), 690–693.

59 Established in the late 1920s, the hospital rendered its services until the mid-1930s and after a brief interruption, it resumed its activity until after the end of the Italian rule in 1941.

60 Assefa Balcha, 'Traditional Medicine in Wallo: Its Nature and History', unpublished MA thesis (Addis Ababa University, 1992), 114.

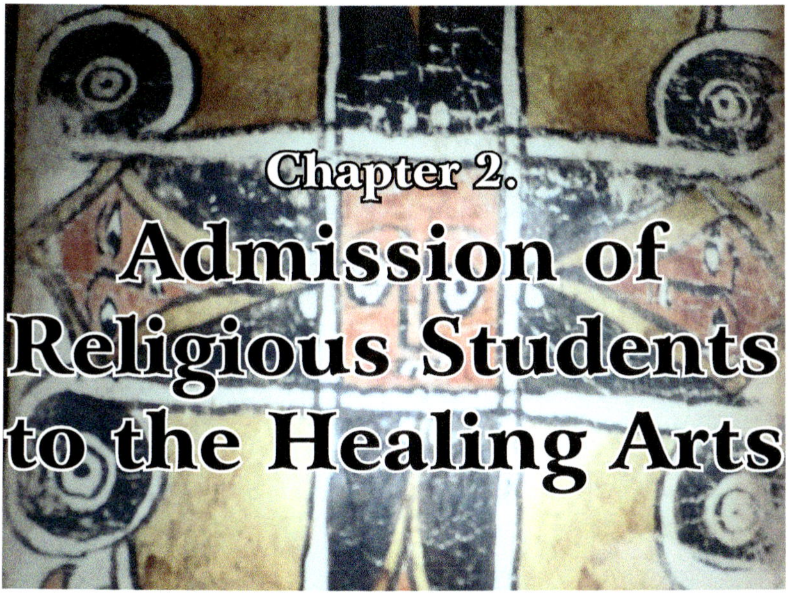

Chapter 2.

Admission of Religious Students to the Healing Arts

At the beginning of the twentieth century, church-based healing dominated the medical landscape of the Amhara region of Ethiopia. This chapter and those that follow examine why this was so. The answer lies, in part, in the relative weakness of other forms of healing, and particularly the inability of Western medicine to mount a serious challenge to church-based healing. The dominance of church-based healing was also based on the overall influence of the Ethiopian Orthodox Tewahedo Church over the people of the region. Yet the power of cleric–healers was also a product of the way in which knowledge of church-based healing was guarded and transmitted to only a few candidates through a lengthy educational process, which included privileged instruction in writing and knowledge of the Ge'ez language.[1] Like physicians in the United States of America during this same period, church-based healers established their claims to medical authority on the basis of their having passed through a rigorous educational process that provided them with privileged access to specialised medical knowledge.

This chapter examines how some religious students developed an interest in church-based medicine, identified cleric–healers, and joined selected religious institutions to learn magico-medical subjects during the 1920s and 1930s. It also discusses the process by which students were selected by cleric–healers for this instruction; and the methods through which future medical students identified religious institutions to learn church-based medical education.

Motivations for Learning Church-based Healing

Students who wanted to become church-based healers, along with other religious students, had to pass through stages of religious learning. Church education normally started at Reading School or the House of Reading (Nebab Bet).[2] Here young students were taught to read and master the Ethiopian alphabet (strictly speaking a syllabary) called the *Fidel*, and memorise a few passages from the Old and New Testaments. After this stage, the road was open for a student either to become a deacon, a priest or to continue learning at a higher level. Students who chose the last-mentioned path would join the first of the three schools of higher learning called the *Zema Bet* (School of Music). The curriculum included the study of *deguwa* (musical notations), Eucharist songs (Zemarie), *mewasit* (songs for commemorations and funerals) and *qedassie* (general liturgy) and, as a synthesis of all, *aquaquam* (religious dance). Mastering all these branches of knowledge normally required eight or more years.

Having completed the Zema Bet, students would join the Qene Bet (School of Poetry), the second stage in the church's pedagogical system of higher learning. Here students studied the Ge'ez *sewasew* (grammar) and the different stages of composing *derset* (religious poetry). Students had to be intelligent enough to withstand the challenges of studying Ge'ez grammar and poetry. The teaching method in this school required students to spend most of their time thinking and producing well-composed and meaningful *qene* verses in Ge'ez. Unlike in other branches of religious learning, to practise and assimilate *qene* lessons was a difficult academic exercise where a student strained 'his power of expression to construct the *qene* verses in a vivid, enigmatic manner or to express his experience in social life in connection with biblical stories, visions, and legendary events'.[3] To become a well-versed *qene* scholar, a student had to spend, on average, a decade learning. The most prestigious *qene* schools were located in the provinces of Wallo and Gojjam.

The third branch of higher learning that required several years of study was Metsehaf Bet (School of the Book). In this school students needed to study several religious and secular texts. Interpretation of the New and Old Testaments, and books on monastic life (*Book of Hermits*), *awald* (apocryphal) texts, and a number of historical and legal tracts, such as the *Kibre Negast* (Glory of Kings), *Fetha Nagast* (Laws of Kings), *Tarika Nagast*) (Chronicles of Kings, *Sirata Mangist* (System of Government), *Bahra Hasab*, *Abushakir* or *Merha Ewur* (the computation of the church calendar) and *physiologus*[4] were studied.

It was in the course of this religious training that students developed a desire to acquire medical knowledge. The motivational factors that pushed religious students to the healing arts varied. However, many were first introduced to the healing arts through the use of *abinet* (education medicines) or memory-enhancing drugs, which they acquired in order to meet the difficult educational demands of ecclesiastical education.[5] The need for education drugs was a particularly pronounced notion among students of *qene* or religious poetry. The difficulty of learning *qene* pushed students to beg for educational *abinet* from their teachers.[6] Students who sought educational *abinet* often experienced trouble with their learning. 'I was not doing well in my studies,' stated an informant, 'and my teacher had given me an educational *abinet* in the form of a magic scroll which made me competitive in some respect, but I wish I had the drug [*abesho*] which could have helped me become an exceptionally intelligent student,'[7] he lamented. Some very intelligent students desired education drugs because they lacked confidence.[8] The desire for educational *abinet*, particularly the inebriating drug called *abesho*, was very strong in students with extraordinary ambition to learn the healing arts, and some of them went to great lengths to obtain the much esteemed *nech abesho* or white *abesho*, which was mostly found among the semi-nomadic peoples of the Nile Valley region. Those who obtained white *abesho*, which purportedly produced the best quality educational *abinet*, were exceedingly lucky.

After taking the memory-boosting drug and passing through a few days of disorientation, a student would show tangible signs of attaining an exceptionally active memory; useful for memorising innumerable religious–magical prayers and texts, along with the names and purposes of hundreds of medicinal items. Educational *abinet* was also said to change naturally timid or nervous students into socially interactive, less fearful, articulate and academically brilliant learners.[9]

Teachers agreed to provide students with educational *abinet* to help them learn ecclesiastical subjects with little pain. Even teachers who had little or no magico-medical training provided students with an ordinary academic *abinet*, a magico-religious prayer intended to help students study and retain religious lessons. Referring probably to this particular educational *abinet,* C. H. Walker, a former British Consul for Western Ethiopia, noted in the early 1930s that some of the professors 'have a medicine which they give to the boys [students] that they may remember well'.[10] Teachers also employed educational *abinet* to recruit students to work with them. A cleric–teacher with a history of high-quality educational *abinet* could attract many students to his site. The experience with educational *abinet* had a strong bearing on students' attitude towards magico-medical subjects and their decision to pursue higher-level ecclesiastical and medical learning.

Although many religious students were attracted to church-based medicine in order to overcome the challenges of learning, students also had other motives for seeking medical training. The desire to overcome particular ailments or disabilities pushed some to learn about medicine. For others it was the need to avenge the death of a family member that led them to the healing arts. The need for personal protection or defence was another reason why students sought out magico-medical wisdom. Yet for others the curiosity of learning about the secrets of the physical and non-physical worlds was an important factor.[11]

For still other students, exposure to small amounts of magico-medical knowledge led them to want to become cleric–healers; for example, one student acquired some magical information after he had told his teacher about the mistreatment that he had received at the hands of religious students in a neighbouring province. The teacher, who was a cleric–healer, was angered by this information and gave the student a few evil spells to avenge his enemies and defend himself in future.[12] The student went on to seek additional medical knowledge. It should be noted, however, that obtaining magico-medical information from a cleric–teacher did not guarantee additional lessons from the same teacher. However, once a student developed an interest in the healing arts, he might well become motivated to gain admission to, and learning church-based medicine from, cleric–teachers working in other religious institutions. Finally, students who acquired a computation of the church calendar magico-medical texts through various ways were also very anxious to learn the healing arts under the tutorship of well-educated cleric–healers.[13]

The decision to pursue further instruction in the healing arts was not without risks or costs. To begin with, church leaders viewed such instructions critically, associating them with the black arts. Other than exalting the supposedly extraordinary medicinal/curative value of 'holy water', the church considered all kinds of medical knowledge satanic.[14] It also rejected the possibility that human actions could bring about cures. Despite church opposition, the quest for *tibeb* (wisdom), a catchword better experienced than defined, was always great, according to cleric–healers. The serious warnings and penalties, for those who pursued magico-medicine, enshrined in the Law of Kings (Fetha Nagast)[15] and the Faith of the Fathers (*Haymanote Abew*)[16] had little impact on those 'convinced seekers of the never-ending earthly wisdoms'.[17] Healers even argued that the quest for wisdom led Adam and Eve to eat the fruit of the forbidden 'tree of knowledge'. Their subsequent death was, in fact, an inevitable price they had to pay for seeking wisdom.[18] It was also common knowledge that those seeking medical knowledge had to trespass beyond the bounds of accepted church knowledge; a requirement that associated church-based healers with the 'black arts' or 'offensive medicine'.[19]

Despite this association and the church's official rejection of the value of religious-based medical knowledge, the church resisted an all-out attack on those who pursued this knowledge and, in fact, turned a blind eye to those who did. This was a largely pragmatic position, based on the recognition that church-based healing was pervasive among the clergy.[20] If the church had taken serious measures against church-based healers, argued informants, it would have lost the majority of its officials and educated members, and this would also have threatened its very existence as a viable institution.[21] In contrast, the church's official rejection of these practices and the presence of written injunctions against them seemed to constrain cleric–healers from disseminating their knowledge in a relaxed and open manner. As a result, the transmission of medical knowledge within the church was cloaked in secrecy.

Choosing to pursue the healing arts also involved personal costs, because it required long years of education during which students had to struggle to find teachers who would accept them as students, and work hard to please them. The work was arduous and required travel to a number of religious institutions.

Students seeking admission to the healing arts began by being accepted for training by an initial cleric–healer. Students could identify potential teachers while studying in the Zema Bet. However, it was in the Qene Bet that learned cleric–healers abounded and students had ample opportunity to pursue the healing arts. Oral informants, who had received their training during this period, stated that it was in the Qene Bet that they were first initiated into the healing profession.[22] This belief was so pervasive that enrolling into the Qene Bet was almost equated to signing up to a 'medical' school; and it was, in fact, the promise of being able to learn medical knowledge that drew many academically competent students to the Qene Bet.[23] Other students were only initiated into the medical arts once they had entered the Metsehaf Bet, the last stage of religious learning.

Gaining Admission

In the 1920s and 1930s learning church-affiliated medicine was, in theory, open to all male students determined to become learned cleric–healers.[24] However, teachers were highly selective about with whom they chose to work. As a result, only a few of the students who strove to acquire healing knowledge were able to do so.

Though students made every effort to make a favourable impression on a would-be cleric–teacher, only a few students succeeded in meeting the requirements that cleric–teachers set for aspiring medical students. Cleric–teachers investigated prospective students in imperceptible and discreet ways, looking for particular qualities in them. To begin with, a cleric–teacher would never accept a student who was from the local region. Students had to come from a distant region so that they would not create competition within the local medical marketplace.[25] In addition, cleric–teachers believed that it was easier to enforce the discipline needed to acquire medical knowledge in students who came from another region. This meant that if a student developed an interest in learning the healing arts while at a school near his home, he would have to leave that school and seek a teacher at some distant institution, if he wished to continue his pursuit of medical knowledge. Among the other qualities that a teacher sought in prospective students were personal conduct and the ability to keep secrets. Above all, cleric–teachers wanted to recruit students who had the potential to learn and the strength to withstand the challenges of religious–medical learning. Mere curiosity in the healing arts would not qualify a student to become a disciple of a cleric–teacher.

Aspiring medical students were expected to offer voluntary 'yeoman's service', ranging from 'performing domestic chores to sharing their daily bread'[26] with their teachers. An oral informant, who had received his training in the 1930s, described his own experience: 'It was through persistent pleading, perseverance and offering labor service for more than a year that I succeeded in convincing my teacher to become his disciple and was able to start learning magical–medical wisdom in a piecemeal manner.'[27] Sometimes, however, absolute obedience and offering labour service to one's teacher was not enough to obtain admission. 'I offered unreserved labour service to my *qene* teacher for almost two years,' another informant lamented, 'but it had very little impact on him. He probably did not appreciate my learning potential, if not my personal conduct. Though it was very difficult to accept this despairing situation, I convinced myself not to expect anything from my teacher and I stuck with him until the end of my religious study a year later.'[28]

In fact, after gaining admission, a student had to obey, respect and maintain agreeable relations with his teacher. The slightest mistake or misunderstanding could obstruct his medical education. Those who found themselves dismissed either due to loss of favour, impoliteness or tardiness had a hard time gaining readmission from the same cleric–teachers.[29] Exhibiting a rigidly ritualised pattern of behaviour and maintaining good relations with one's teacher was an essential requirement for anyone wishing to pass through the doorway to the healing arts.

While students were normally chosen on the basis of their character and abilities, some students succeeded in establishing relationships with healers in other ways. A student stricken by sickness and nursed back to health by a cleric–healer could develop a close relationship with him and go on to become his student. In like fashion, physically disabled students, by virtue of the sympathy they enjoyed from their cleric–teachers, might be accorded special privileges and be recruited to learn the healing arts with relative ease. Many cleric–healers were, in fact, disabled. Yet even in these cases, cleric–healers imposed rigorous criteria in evaluating their future students.

Cleric–healers reiterated that physically disabled students, notably visually impaired ones, were particularly well suited to be taught the secrets of magical *abinet*. Since the physically disabled did not qualify to serve as priests, they often took the *dabtara* path, a thoroughfare that helped them become well-educated persons in medico-medical fields.[30] Though the church always viewed disability as a manifestation of God's wrath upon wrongdoers, it did not prevent the physically disabled from joining religious schools; and many disabled individuals were able to pursue higher-level ecclesiastical and medical education.[31] The proverbial belief in the extraordinary learning potential of the visually impaired reflected the belief that their disability made them 'naturally disciplined' and made them especially sympathetic to the troubles of other human beings.[32]

The disabled were also believed to be particularly skilled at keeping secrets and using *abinet* ethically. In addition, they were thought to have an unparalleled ability to memorise magico-medical prayers and prescriptions (even to the point of making ከርታስ or written records worthless).[33]

Oral informants also claimed that disabled students who became healers made excellent teachers. Disabled teachers were considered repositories of both white and black *abinet*, and many able-bodied students approached them to serve as their teachers.[34]

While gaining acceptance by a healer was essential to acquiring medical knowledge, a student also had to excel at his religious studies and particularly in his mastery of the language Ge'ez, which was critical to both medical and religious training. A student who was a slow learner of Ge'ez would not progress fast in his medical education. As a result, the duration of a student's medical–magical education was commensurate with the amount of effort he put in in learning the language. The importance of learning Ge'ez also meant that students sought out teachers who were located at educational institutions that were known for teaching the language.[35]

Expanding One's Knowledge

While students might begin their medical education at one institution, becoming a well-trained cleric–healer necessitated the acquisition of knowledge from a number of teachers located at different institutions.[36] Attachment to a single and well-educated *qene* teacher for a couple of years might be enough for a student to grasp Ge'ez grammar, to compose excellent religious poetry or *qene* and to obtain diverse sorts of medical–magical knowledge. Students who chose to spend five or more years in a particular *qene* or Metsehaf Bet might have forged a long-lasting attachment to a single teacher and obtained a consolidated medical education, but it would be a mistake to assume that staying at a particular place for years would guarantee a medical student in-depth medical–magical knowledge needed to become a healer. This was because while the medical–magical–divinatory knowledge taught by teachers in different churches and monasteries was similar in form, it was different in quality and depth. It was widely acknowledged that no one teacher, no matter how extensive his medical knowledge and collection of medical–magical texts may have been, could provide an aspiring student with the full breadth of available religious medical knowledge. Students were therefore bound to seek out several teachers, often travelling great distances to seek further knowledge.[37]

The need to seek knowledge from several teachers was also dictated by other factors. To begin with, the best teachers attracted many students, each of whom competed to become the teacher's disciple. Students often had to wait long periods in order to be admitted as a disciple of a talented cleric–healer. Impatience could lead a student to move on to another teacher. Thus, one informant described how '[i]n the course of my travels I made two brief sojourns and found that all the teachers with whom I wanted to attach myself were surrounded by students waiting to be admitted as medical students, and I wondered whether I should move on to other teachers before it was too late; which I finally did.'[38]

In addition, acquiring medical knowledge from a cleric–teacher did not follow a set curriculum that could be completed in a clearly defined period. Teachers imparted their knowledge as they saw fit. The pace at which the teacher revealed his knowledge varied greatly and was based on the character of the relationship that a student had with his teacher. Related to this was the fact that the character of the relationship could vary over time, depending on how hard the student worked to please his mentor. In some cases a student who established a strong relationship with a healer might complete his education in a short period. Thus one informant noted, 'I had the privilege to become closer to my teacher who was willing to recruit me to the healing arts; and he taught me considerable magico-medical lessons in about eighteen months. Had it not been for his openness and down-to-earth instructional methods, the amount of knowledge I gathered during this time might have required me to seek repeated admissions and work with three or more teachers for a number of years.'[39] In contrast, some teachers were reluctant to impart all their knowledge to their students and were very slow to reveal what they knew. Teachers could also become displeased with their student's performance and decide to withhold information or slow the educational process. The duration of a student's medical–magical learning was also commensurate with the amount of effort he put in to assimilate Ge'ez, an indispensable prerequisite to learn advanced religious and medical–magical lessons. As a result, a student might have to remain attached to a single teacher for years. Again, impatience led some students to give up hope of learning what they wanted to know from a particular teacher and to seek knowledge elsewhere.[40] As a consequence of these various factors, students hoping to master the healing arts spent years moving from one teacher to another.

Departing from a specific learning site inaugurated a new phase in the pursuit of additional religious and medical learning. At this crucial juncture, medical students had to obtain the blessing of the cleric–teacher they were leaving. Failure to do so could anger that teacher, causing him to punish the departing student for failing to honour or acknowledge his moral and intellectual authority. It was believed that with a powerful magic hex, a slighted cleric–teacher could invalidate the knowledge of a student who had displeased him. This serious measure, which brought about personality disorders, notably insanity or permanent loss of memory, expressed a teacher's resentment against 'ingrate students' who believed that they owed their success, not to their considerate teachers, but to their own personal efforts and abilities.[41]

In choosing additional training sites, religious students always considered the presence of a predominantly Orthodox Christian population that would support and honour religious students (the future 'father confessors' of the faithful) and the suitability of the climate to their health. As noted above, students had to select teachers who were located at some distance away from their homes. As a result, students were obliged to travel from one province to another; for example, a student from Wallo had to travel to Gojjam, Gondar and Shewa. Learning where to find an excellent teacher was not difficult, for while cleric–teachers refused to tell their students about other teachers out of concern for preserving their own reputation or authority, students could learn of potential sites from colleagues coming from the different parts of the Amhara region.[42]

Students did not need to obtain their medical knowledge from different institutions by themselves. Groups of closely connected students could pool their knowledge. Each friend would go to a designated church or monastery and enlist as a medical student of a knowledgeable cleric–healer. After gathering diverse medical–magical information for a year or two, or even up to four years, the team members would reunite at a particular location to share their findings.[43] This group effort greatly helped students reduce the time and energy they needed to devote to studying church-affiliated medicine.

Very popular destinations for religious students looking for educators of medico-magical wisdom were Gojjam (various places), Shewa (especially Manz), Wallo (i.e., Amhara Sayint, Wadla, Lasta, Sokota) and Gondar (quite a number of places in both the North and South). They were also known for teaching top-quality Ge'ez, *qene* and medical–magical matters.[44] The history of religious institutions known for the best-quality education was intertwined with that of famous cleric–teachers imparting magico-medical lessons. Many informants believed that more than the history of religious institutions per se, the presence of cleric–teachers made some churches and monasteries famous;[45] for example, the unbroken presence of highly educated teachers in the various *qene* schools in Gojjam gave rise to a very popular legend linking Gojjam to the beginning of church-affiliated medicine and healing.

The arduous quest for medical knowledge, entailing years of service to various cleric–healers, did not always lead to a successful ending. Many students, failing to develop strong relationships with well-known cleric–healers, developed only a partial knowledge of the medical arts. Some gave up the quest. As a result, the number of healers who could claim to have mastered church-based medical knowledge was considerably smaller than the number of students who sought this knowledge. This selection process contributed to the respect and authority that fully trained healers enjoyed in the medical marketplace. The next chapter will examine in more detail the educational process through which medical knowledge was conveyed and the nature of that knowledge.

Figure 6: Talismanic drawing inserted in a magico-religious protective amulet

Source: Courtesy of IES

Figure 7: A personal amulet to fight against malevolent spiritual entities

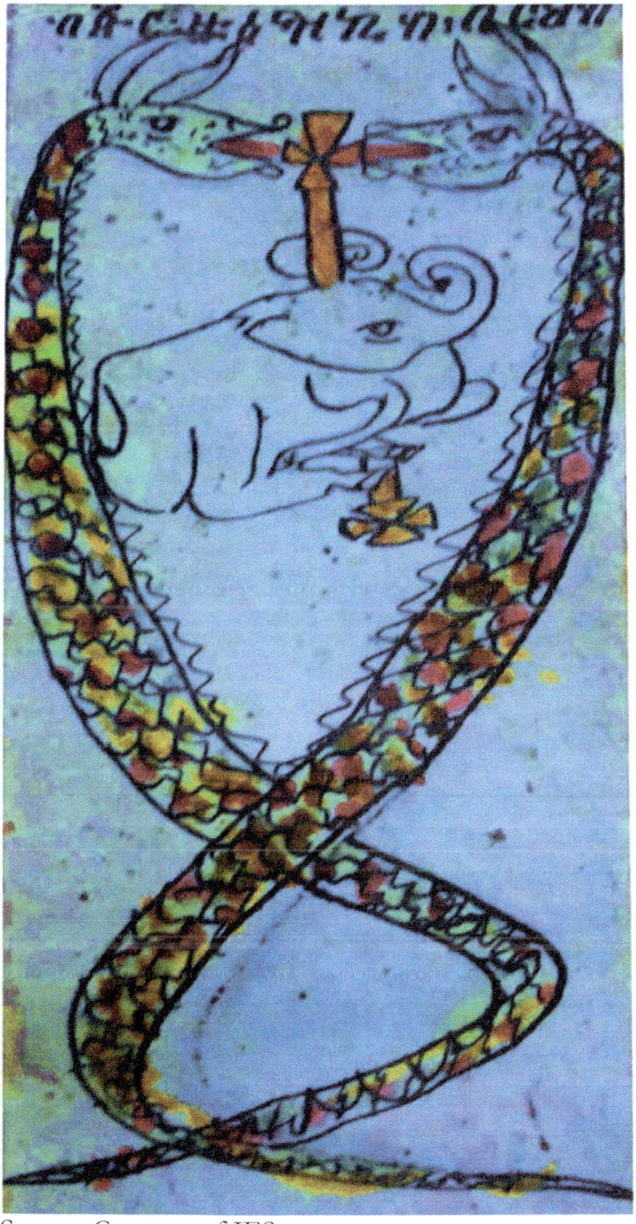

Source: Courtesy of IES

Notes

1 Ge'ez as a 'consecrated' language has also been referred to as the 'language of prophecy', the 'tongue of the Angels' and the 'first language of Adam and Eve'. Leykun Berhanu, *Remorse* (Amharic) (Addis Ababa: Neged Printing Press), 6–11.

2 For a brief discussion of the four-tiered school system of the Orthodox Church, see Inbaqom Qalawold, *Traditional Ethiopian Church Education*, translated into English by Mengistu Lemma (New York: Teachers' College Press, 1970). For a detailed pedagogical account, see Habte Mariam Workneh, *Ethiopian Traditional Education* (Addis Ababa: Berhanena Selam Printing Press, 1962 E.C.); also see Kidane Mariam Getahun, *The Traditional Ethiopian Student* (Amharic) (Addis Ababa: Tensae Zagubae Printing Press, 1954 E.C.).

3 The Ethiopian Orthodox Church, *The Ethiopian Church*, 94.

4 Oral informants nos. 9, 15, 18, 19, 22, 23, 27, 30, 33 and 37. *Physiologus* was a work of the second or third century CE on the natural history of animals, plants and minerals. The book is believed to have been originally written in Greek and interpreted into Ge'ez.

5 Educational *abinet* or የቀለም አብነት constituted አብሾ, ዕፀ ፋርስ, አጠፋሪስ or አስተናግር[5] (*abesho*, *etse fars* or *atafaris*, *astanagir*), and various compositions of magic prayer or አስማት (*asmat*) such as ዘኢ.ያገድፍ ('to support' or 'to assist'), and አፍልሆ *afliho*, a cup of sanctified holy water that would bubble when resins were included. See Marcel Griaule, Griaule, Marcel. 'Mythes, croyances et coutumes de Begameder (Abyssinie), *Journal Asiatique* (1928): 65; IES, Ms. No. 2244; Jacques Mercier, 'Les hallucinogenes ethiopiens identification', *Abbay* 10 (1979); also Wallis Budge, *Bandlet of Righteousness: An Ethiopian Book of the Dead* (London: Luzac & Co., 1929).

6 *Qene* is defined as 'የተማሪውን ሰውነት እንደቅንቅን እንደነቀዝ የሚጎዳ' (literally 'It is just like earworm and weevil that damages a student's body'), Desta Tekle Wold, *New Amharic Dictionary*, 1079.

7 Oral informant no. 14; for example, licking off a magic prayer inscribed on both sides of a sharpened sword would help a student become an extraordinarily intelligent learner. To exorcise ኢይነጥላ, a spirit that held students back from learning fast was a common practice. See Wallis Budge, *Bandlet of Righteousness*, pp. 3–12. Teachers also provided specifically targeted magical prayers to their students, such as to improve their writing or reading skill, for learning religious poetry or music, and the list goes on. See IES, Ms. No. 2244. In this manuscript one finds a phrase: ለዝንቱ፡ መጽሐፍ ዘወጽአ በዘመነ ባካፋ ንጉሰ ነገስት (lit. 'This

text [of educational *abinet*] was produced [in the eighteenth century] during the reign of Emperor Bakaffa').

8 Oral informants nos. 20, 21 and 27.

9 Ibid.

10 C. H. Walker, *The Abyssinian at Home* (London, 1933), 12. For a list of written educational *abinet*, see Girmay Berhane, 'The Dabtara Doctor Asmat' (Amharic), unpublished BA thesis (Haile Selassie I University, 1970), 11.

11 Oral informants nos. 4, 11, 23, 33 and 39; the love of wisdom has been expressed in the dictum: ጥበብ ይኄይስ እም ብዙኅ መዛግብት (literally 'Wisdom is much better than a large collection of written records'). Even the celibates, who had very little earthly interests, were no exception to this rule, informants commented.

12 Oral informant no. 36.

13 Oral informants nos. 31 and 35.

14 Holy water 'sanctifies whoever is touched by it, frees him from uncleanness, and attacks the power of darkness, and secures that wherever it is sprinkled there is freedom from pestilence and snares of Satan'. See Aymro Wondmageghehu and Joachim Motovu (eds), *The Ethiopian Orthodox Church* (Addis Ababa: The Ethiopian Orthodox Mission, 1970), 72.

15 The Ethiopian Orthodox Church, *Fetha Nagast* (Amharic and Ge'ez) (Addis Ababa: Berhanena Selam Printing Press, 1958 E.C.), 544: the book dealing with ecclesiastical and earthly matters, known to have been written under the auspices of Constantine the Great and introduced to Ethiopia by way of Coptic Egypt during the reign of Zara Yaqob (1414–1468) and translated into Ge'ez. It was used as a legal code of the country until its total replacement with the Penal Code in 1930 and the Civil Code in 1960.

16 The Ethiopian Orthodox Church, *Haymanote Abew* [The Faith of the Fathers] (Amharic) (Addis Ababa: Tensae Zagubae Printing Press, 1986 E.C.), 591–92; This book, a compendium of the works of several scholars of the Eastern Orthodox Church, allegedly translated from Arabic to *Geez* and published in Amharic in 1975 after reviewed by the Intellectual Council of the Ethiopian Orthodox Church.

17 Oral informant no. 27.

18 Oral informants nos. 20, 33 and 39; craving for wisdom should not necessarily be subordinated to the idea of damnation, argued informants, for '[i]t is not enough for the human race to live on earth and to produce and reproduce *sui generis*; it would be wise to examine and understand the secrets of nature and to decide its own fate . . . which would be expressed in revealing the unseen, reading the

unrecorded, concealing the printed, defeating the undefeatable, etc.' Zenebe Abraha, *Spirits* (Amharic) (Addis Ababa: Berhanena Selam Printing Press, 1992 E.C.), 33–35.

19 Oral informants nos. 2, 4, 30 and 38. 'Though the church officially frowns on it,' writes Weissleder, 'many priests are known to have such knowledge and ability, and to use it at will . . . [t]hey are feared . . . by the members of their own church community . . . even the heads of churches treat these men with all the deference that will insure their benevolence.' See Wolfgang Weissleder, 'The Political Ecology of Amhara Domination'. Unpublished PhD dissertation (University of Chicago, 1965), 78.

20 Oral informants nos. 12, 21, 30 and 57.

21 Oral informants nos. 4, 11, 12, 18, 20, 21 and 35.

22 Oral informants nos. 12, 20, 21 and 22.

23 The notion of associating medical learning with *qene* scholars has resonated in an oral tradition of the sixteenth century, which would probably justify the time–depth of Ethiopian church-based medicine and healing.

24 Ecclesiastical education was restricted to men.

25 It was not only to avoid future competition in the trade, but also to protect them from any sort of magical attack from former students (either out of jealousy or in the service of clients) that cleric–healers did not want to negotiate on the issue of teaching students coming from nearby districts or provinces.

26 Oral informants nos. 18, 26 and 39.

27 Oral informant no. 37.

28 Oral informant no. 57.

29 Oral informants nos. 2, 19, 20, 22 and 31.

30 Johnny Bakke, *Christian Ministry: Patterns and Functions Within the Ethiopian Evangelical Church Mekane Yesus* (New Jersey: Humanities Press, 1987), 72.

31 A disabled person gaining a measure of religious and medico-magical knowledge could easily escape from becoming a beggar or a burden to society. The visually and physically disabled, not to mention those with multiple disabilities, were the two major congenital types of disability commonly seen in religious schools; for instance, a cleric–healer who prepared a voluminous medical text noted that he obtained the sympathy of his teacher when he was poisoned by his colleagues around the late 1930s; being outraged by what had happened to the student, the teacher acquiesced to teaching him medicine. See Biniam Weldegebreil, 'Traditional Medicine Practitioners of Addis Ababa: A

Historical Account from Imperial Times to the Present', unpublished BA thesis (Addis Ababa University, 1998), 7–9.

32 Being victims of disability, they would not easily be tempted to misuse their medico-magical knowledge at whim. It was also widely believed that due to some mistakes in applying the techniques of conjuring evil spirits that many previously healthy *dabtara* became physically handicapped.

33 Oral informants nos. 32, 36, 44, and 55.

34 Oral informants nos. 10, 33, 37 and 57.

35 Oral informants are unanimous on this idea.

36 Temesgen Gebre, *Autobiography* (Amharic) (Addis Ababa: Alpha Printers, 2001 E.C.), 19ff. According to Feierman, healers involved in individual cures were also required to travel widely to collect medical knowledge. Steven Feierman, *Peasant Intellectuals, Anthropology and History in Tanzania*, (Madison: University of Wisconsin Press, 1990), 103.

37 Temesgen Gebre, *Autobiography*, 19ff.

38 Oral informant no. 30.

39 Oral informant no. 42.

40 A student from Gondar had to work with half-a-dozen teachers in Shewa and Wallo before he became a fully-fledged cleric–healer. Oral informant no. 4. Another student from Gayint (south Gondar) first went to Manz (north Shewa) and studied medico-magical and divinatory lessons for about 12 years, and then he moved to Dawint and Wadla (both in north Wallo) and did the same for 3 and 2 years respectively. Oral informant no. 21.

41 Oral informants nos. 12, 19, 27, 30 and 44; the magic spell cleric–healers employed for this particular purpose was known as አስማት፡ መፍዝዝ ወመቅዝዝ አስማት መፍዝዝ ወመደንግዝ (literally 'A magic spell employed to make a person indolent and unproductive').

42 Oral informants nos. 19, 27, 35, 39, 44.

43 Oral informants nos. 2, 10, 11, 12, 13, 17, 18, 20, 22, 26, 35 and 39. For the pervasiveness of this learning strategy in much of the twentieth century, see Alemayehu Moges, 'Traditional Ethiopian Medicine,' *8th International Conference of Ethiopian Studies*, volume I (Addis Ababa, 1984), 117–118.

44 During the twentieth century Gonj and Washera in Gojjam and Wadla in Wallo were highly acclaimed for their *qene* schools and medical education. Places such as Debra Libanos and Debra Birhan in Shewa (including some churches in Addis Ababa); Bethlehem, Deresge Maryam, Mahbere Selassie, Qomma Fasiladas, Zuramba, and Mekane Iyasus in north and south Gondar; Martole Maryam, Dima Giyorgis, Debra Worq, Qaranyo, Yews, Elias, Dangera, Washera, Gonj, Debra

Mawi, Wura, Geshe Abbay in Gojjam were also prominent for the study of *qene*, the Scriptures, law (or *Fetha Negast*), and Bahra Hasab. Tadbaba Maryam, Atronsa Maryam, Meskaba Qeddusan, Qarana Maryam, Afqara Qirqos, and some other monasteries in places such as Lalibela, Sokota and Hayq were also eminent places of book learning. In the same vein, Zuramba in Begemdir and Selal Kula in Wallo were well-known for church music. See Inbaqom Qala Wold, 'Traditional Ethiopian Church Education', (Amharic) *Proceeding of the Third International Conference on Ethiopian Studies*, vol. 2 (Addis Ababa: Institute of Ethiopian Studies, Haile Selassie I University, 1969), 11–33; Alemayehu Moges, 'The Traditional Church Education,' unpublished BTh thesis (Holy Trinity Theological College, 1971), 10–11; Habte Mariam Workneh, *The Traditional Ethiopian Curriculum* (Amharic) (Addis Ababa: Berhanena Selam Printing Press, 1962 E.C.), 101, 285–287.

45 Oral informants nos. 12, 22, 24, 26, 29, 35 and 39.

Chapter 3. Learning Church-based Medical Education

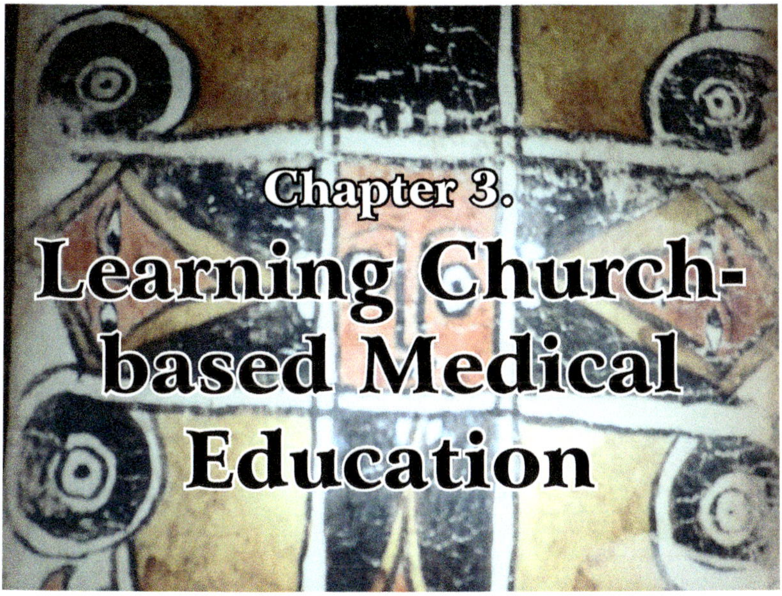

This chapter attempts to look more closely at the arduous process by which religious students in the Orthodox Church learnt to be cleric–healers. Students interested in pursuing the healing arts had to identify teachers, while teachers, on their part, had to evaluate them for admission. In order to be admitted, students needed to demonstrate their commitment to a teacher by providing menial services. These services continued once a student had been accepted for medical training. They were a kind of tuition that included gathering wood for the master's fire, tilling his garden, washing his clothes, washing his feet and those of his guests, pounding grain, cooking food, and performing other domestic chores.[1] Students were also expected to provide for themselves and their teacher while studying ecclesiastical subjects. To do this, they travelled hours begging for scraps of bread or injera[2] from the surrounding villages.[3] The service demands were particularly high for those students who chose to work with disabled teachers.

Students moved from teacher to teacher in order to complete their medical training. The willingness and speed with which a teacher conveyed his knowledge to a student was dependent upon the student's continued proper conduct, and willingness to discharge his moral and ethical responsibilities.[4] Failing to demonstrate unwavering adherence to the teacher's will could lead to dismissal or a slowdown in a student's education. Having said this, this chapter will make clear the actual educational process through which medical knowledge was imparted to would-be medical students.

Learning Magico-Religious and Magico-Medical Subjects

After obtaining admission to the healing arts, aspiring medical students were confronted with the challenges of mastering the spiritual and non-spiritual aspects of church-based medical education. The spiritual side constituted magico-religious and magico-medical subjects. In principle, magico-religious knowledge included practices that were permissible from the perspective of the church, while magico-medical knowledge involved the use of the black arts and were viewed by the church as non-permissible. In actual practice, however, the line between these two categories of knowledge was not so clear. Thus slight alterations of permissible prayers, for example, could transform them into non-permissible prayers that bordered on magico-medical practice. In effect, there were three categories of knowledge that a student healer needed to master: (1) permissible magico-religious knowledge, which was required of all clerical students; (2) non-permissive magico-religious, which bordered on the black arts; and (3) magico-medical knowledge, which constituted the black arts.

Magico-Religious Prayers

Access to magico-religious knowledge was open to almost all ecclesiastical students. One of the foremost duties of religious students was to learn about magico-religious texts known by the generic name *yastelote metsehaft* (prayer books), alias *digam* (prayers) not *digimt* (evil magic prayers or spells). Prayer texts were mostly prepared by taking some passages from the Bible, the litanies of the Mass, and devotional books of various angels, martyrs and saints[5] and, of course, from apocryphal or extrabiblical and other texts where the secret names of Jesus and the Almighty have been found to abound.[6] The principal object of reciting prayer texts was to help a person solicit uninterrupted protection from benevolent spiritual entities, to fight off or keep away evil spirits and, ultimately, to lead a healthier life free from spiritual and physical ordeals.

For many physical illnesses and social difficulties, the *dersan* (homilies) and *malk* (images) composed in the name of the Almighty/Holy Trinity, the archangels, saints, martyrs, biblical and apocryphal figures, monastic holy men, the insignia of the church,[7] sacred days and liturgical ideas were widely employed as preventative and therapeutically important magico-religious prayers. Magico-religious prayers such as Temherta Hebuat[8] (Lessons on Mystery), Asmata Malakot (lit. 'Secret Names of Divinity'), *Mashafa Tuladan* (*Book of Tuladan*, a compendium of prayers to solicit deference and protection from the evil influence of destructive powers) and *Mashafa Bartos* (*Book of Bartos*, a collection of prayers of Saint Mary at a place called *Bartos*) were mostly used for keeping evil demons at bay.[9]

Other prayers were simply identified by their alleged purposes or the names of the disease they claimed to ward off or defeat. Tselota Nadera (Prayer Against Nadera) and Tselota Aynatila (Prayer Against Aynatila) were vital magico-religious prayers to fight against the evil eye or an illness resembling the evil eye. While Lessane Sab[10] was intended to fight against backbiters or malediction, Sayfa Malakot (Sword of the Divinity)[11] and Sayfa Selassie (Sword of the Trinity)[12] were acknowledged as having considerable protective value. Magico-religious texts that contained non-offensive prayers also included **መጽሐፈ ፈውስ መንፈሳዊ** (*Book of Spiritual Therapy*), **መጽሐፈ አስማት ጥሩ ጥሩ** (*Book of Prayers with Benign Intent*), **መጽሐፈ ጥበብ** (*Book of Wisdom*) or simply as **መጽሐፈ ፀሎት መድሐኒተ ነፍስ ወሥጋ** (*Book of Prayer: A Panacea for the Body and Soul*).[13]

One of the underlining concepts in the preparation of an endless variety of magico-religious prayers has been the use of *asmat* or secret names of the Creator from whom His mother, Mary, and the archangels were said to have obtained the power to perform miracles.[14] By examining a magico-religious text called *Arde'et*, Enno Littmann has shown the various secret names and attributes of Jesus Christ.[15] A similar method was utilised in the production of magico-religious prayers composed in the name of the archangels and several holy figures.[16] Despite the underlying commonality linking magico-religious prayers, they can be grouped into four major categories: (1) prayers in the name of the Almighty; (2) angels and holy figures (i.e., saints, martyrs and prophets); and those of (3) sacred ideas; and (4) sacred objects.

Magico-religious prayers were mostly recited by inserting the patients' baptismal names so as to help them regain their health.[17] They were intended to fight against a number of illnesses and personal or social mishaps.[18] Since disease-causing spirits were not precisely identified, these prayers were viewed as combating a myriad of noxious spirits. Many magico-religious texts were also recited to consecrate the therapeutically efficacious *tabal* or holy water,[19] in which a patient was often immersed.[20]

Although the great majority of magico-religious prayers were viewed as permissible by the church, many others were not. Access to, and mastery of, non-permissible prayers was what distinguished ecclesiastic or cleric–healers from the majority of the mainstream clergy.[21] To protect the secret of their 'success' and to avoid criticism, cleric–healers were careful not to reveal their non-permissible magical prayers to others.[22]

Magico-Medical Knowledge (Non-Permissible Prayers)

When one looks at non-permissible magico-religious prayers, they appear similar to the purely religious, well-intentioned or sacred prayers. Like permissible prayers, almost all non-permissible prayers begin with the phrase: 'In the name of the Father and the Son and the Holy Spirit one Divinity prayer against . . . ' and cite names of benevolent spiritual figures. They thus appear to be 'religious' and permissible. However, they are 'profane' because they contain several secret names, 'words and phrases of power', and *gabir* (instructions) on their manner of application, including chants, actions and gestures, as well as substances needed to achieve their intended results.[23] The insertion of these magical words and instructions transformed acceptable religious prayers into non-sanctioned magical practices that were condemned by the church. From the cleric–healer's perspective, magico-religious prayers only achieved their desired results when used in combination with their *gabir*.[24] That is why a student of the healing arts spent a great deal of time learning about the intended purpose and manner of application, *gabir*, of non-permissible magico-religious prayers.

It was widely believed that the practice of beginning with the phrase: 'In the name of the Father and the Son and the Holy Spirit' in non-permissible magical prayers began during the reign of Emperor Zara Yaqob (1434–1468), a period of 'Ethiopian literary renaissance' in which an extensive body of religious and non-religious (i.e., divinatory and apocryphal) texts were known to have been translated into Ge'ez.[25] Before that time, non-permissible prayers started with various names for the devil, or other maleficent spirits. The emperor, being fearful of 'spirits and sorcerers',[26] ordered his agents to wipe out all occult literature and practices.[27] To confound Zara Yaqob's agents, the clerics lost no time in inserting the phrase: 'In the name of the Father and the Son and the Holy Spirit' in the very first line of all non-permissive magical prayers.[28]

Acquiring Magico-Religious Knowledge

Students who created strong contacts with cleric teachers were able to learn non-permissive prayers and their proper administration through the reading of magico-religious texts secretly kept by their teachers.[29] To do so, they had to obtain the requisite copying skills and permission of their teacher. Accessing magical prayers without a teachers' permission was a totally unacceptable act; for example, a student assigned as a copyist by his teacher would not dare to make unauthorised copies. No matter how accomplished a student might be, he must not appear to be acting on his own; and any such action would amount to besmirching his teacher.

Nonetheless, students sometime stole texts from a teacher in order to save time and eliminate the enormous travail that he would normally need to go through in order to gain access to the knowledge found in the text.[30] The student would then seek out another teacher in a faraway location who could interpret the text for him. In return, the new teacher would expand his own knowledge and collection of texts.[31]

This undesirable behaviour is understandable when one considers that only a few students were able to learn church-based medicine, while other students had to wait indefinitely, hoping that they might be accepted some day.[32] Impatience with waiting indefinitely pushed some students to take illegal action, such as stealing teachers' medico-magical texts.[33] One aged informant remembered a case from around the time of the Italian occupation in which a student had stolen a medico-magical text and an educational *abinet* from his teacher.[34] The student had exhausted his patience with waiting indefinitely, while some of his colleagues had obtained educational *abinet* from the same teacher.[35]

Such acts of dishonesty were condemned by most cleric–healers, who admonished their students to live honest lives. Stressing the potential drawbacks and the price to be paid for exhibiting malicious characteristics such as dishonesty, thievery and other undesirable deeds, cleric teachers frequently told their students to humbly yield up their lives to a higher cause.[36] Students were even told not to crib the *qene* (or poems) of other scholars;[37] and it was in keeping with these conceptual rules that cleric teachers sought to cultivate their disciples and sustain what might be dubbed a kind of 'clerical underworld'.

To closely guard the secrets of their magico-medical texts and to discourage students from engaging in unwanted behaviours, such as the indiscriminate use of offensive or harmful magic spells,[38] many cleric–healers translated their texts into a kind of code created by applying a writing technique known as *nagara dabtara* (*dabtara*'s affair).[39] In this highly technical writing or stenographic method cleric teachers employed one or more of the following tricks: substituting words with numbers; using incomplete or shortened words or phrases; substituting syllables or words with different syllables or words; using abbreviated words, phrases or obscure nomers; putting magical prayers and their applications separately; writing parts of a prayer from right to left instead of the usual left to right; changing the place of words in a sentence or a paragraph; misplacing syllables in a word or phrase; inscribing part of a prayer in one page and the remaining part in a different page; writing therapeutic instructions partly in Ge'ez and partly in Amharic; and inscribing complete prayers with incomplete *gabir* or manner of application.[40] Acquiring medico-magical knowledge from texts containing *nagara dabtara* was extremely difficult, and even if a student succeeded in breaking the code, he might not be able to unearth all the concealed information it contained.[41] 'It is just like having *injera* [a pancake like preparation] without *wot* [a peppery stew],' noted an informant.[42] The use of *nagara dabtara*, therefore, ensured that medical students could only access the hidden knowledge contained in medico-magical texts through the goodwill and acquiescence of their cleric teachers.

Navigating the complexities of *nagara dabtara*, was only one of the roles that teachers played in educating medical students on the complexity of magico-religious texts. Students were also closely monitored and instructed on abstract Ge'ez concepts, while studying magico-medical texts.[43] They were also instructed in the benefits and potential drawbacks of written *abinet*, and the importance of internalising all the information communicated to them through what may be called 'assign–study–recite formula' of instruction.[44] Students were continually warned against the temptation to plunge prematurely into experimenting with prayers and *abinet*. In a situation where most instructions comprised very complex rituals, including the invocation of noxious spiritual beings, students had to keep themselves away from an 'undirected immersion' in magical experimentations.[45] While students were encouraged to carry out some experimentation under the watchful eyes of their teachers, they were constantly reminded 'to show considerable self-restraint from any perilous trial or rehearsal' or not to take a single step on their own.[46] Those who did not observe these procedures would put themselves and others at risk.

Magico-Medical Knowledge, Learning the Black Arts

The aspiration to become a well-educated cleric–diviner persuaded many students to develop an interest in *yakefat abinet,* or offensive medicine that was totally separate from church-based permissive or non-permissive prayers. The church associated *Yakefat abinet* with evil and it constituted what could be called the *black arts*. So, how could students of the healing arts learn about and acquire these evil-intended prayers?

To gain access to, and learn about, evil magic spells was a cumbersome experience. Almost all information about the black arts was jealously guarded; and a student with an interest in evil magic had to go through an extended 'waiting period' and satisfy characteristically distinct evaluation criteria set by his teacher(s). Jacques Mercier, noting the scarcity of magic spells, says '*Dans tout le domaine de la magie noire il est extremement rare de trouver un manuscrit ancien*'

(Throughout the field of black magic it is extremely rare to find an ancient manuscript).[47]

A student with an interest in offensive medicine had to obtain the permission of his teacher to learn harmful or black magic. This permission was only granted to a select few students of high character. Teachers tried to prevent students who were mean spirited and who might use the knowledge for vengeful purposes or to achieve economic benefit from gaining access to knowledge of the black arts, because it was widely believed that its use by such students would bring total disgrace to themselves and to the healing profession.

In selecting students to learn the black arts, teachers applied different criteria from those used in selecting medical students in general. Students selected the black arts needed to demonstrate unflinching discipline, self-cultivation, and unfailing interest in learning this highly secret and sinister knowledge. In addition, cleric–teachers strongly preferred students born under the sign of Mizan Nafas or Libra, the seventh Zodiac.[48] A Mizan Nafas person was known for his extraordinary open-mindedness, his ability to retain power, and his potential to become a distinguished scholar and healer.[49] Such persons were seen as particularly well suited to all medical training, but when it came to selecting students for the black arts, few non-Mizan Nafas students were chosen.[50]

Evil–magical spells were employed to bring about scores of illnesses, including incurable and debilitating ones, insanity and even sudden death. There were also numerous magico-medical prayers that were aimed at specific villainous targets, such as striking at the foundations of marriages or inter-personal relationships.[51] Magico-medical prayers were also viewed as more effective in earning money, favour, respect, love (from authorities or the opposite sex) and other privileges than permissible magico-religious prayers.[52] As long as similar techniques were used (e.g., charms and amulets) in both helpful (medical or protective) and harmful magic prayers, the difference between the two lay not in their basic conception but in the purposes they served or 'the means used'.[53]

Evil magical prayers can be found in abundance in Manuscript No. 2417 of the Institute of Ethiopian Studies library, a compendium of manuscripts of 2 639 pages. This manuscript contains several varieties of magico-medical prayers directed against illnesses, personal or social problems.[54] This compilation undoubtedly required the co-operation of cleric–healers who collected prayers over many decades.

Sinister magical prayers could be prepared and applied in a wide variety of ways. However, these prayers shared certain common characteristics. To begin with, magic spells and incantations were particularly effective if Satan, alias *Satnael* or *Diablos*, the supreme evil spirit, and his subordinates, the demons, were properly invoked. The demon's name was recited together with the name of the intended victim.[55] The legend of Satnael,[56] being a source of evil wisdom, provided cleric–healers with the impetus to defy God's laws, and to acquire and perform magical wonders using the virtues and vices of Satnael.[57]

Successfully invoking the power of Satan and his demons required healers to enter into a relationship with them. This was a highly dangerous act. The procedure for establishing friendship with evil-spirits was referred to as መዋረስ *mawares* (inheritance).[58] *Mawares* was a very scary experience which would expose 'human partners to pathogenic attacks from evil spirits'. This act also 'evoked divine displeasure because it involved seeking power and knowledge beyond the limits of the moral order'.[59] A person avidly interested in befriending the devil (and in mastering demon-conjuring skills) had to renounce Christ, The Prince of Peace, and the Orthodox faith, and he had to go through a period of fasting and reciting prayers composed in the name of Satnael, known universally as መልክአ ሳጥናኤል *Malka Satnael* (Image of Satnael) and ድርሳነ ሳጥናኤል *Dersana Satnael* (Homily of Satnael).[60] With the help of these prayers and associated rituals, notably shedding the blood of a sheep or a black fowl, sprinkling home-made alcoholic drinks such as *taj*, *talla* and *araqi*, brewing coffee and burning incense and other aromatic items such as *karbe*, *altit*, *wogart*, and *taj sar*,[61] a person secluded for a week 'inherited' Satnael and became a 'demon puller'. However, this process could be fatal. Thus an elderly healer noted, 'I had two friends, the one who succeeded in "inheriting" and conjuring up the devil, and the other one killed by the devil while performing the ritual on his way to becoming a demon puller.'[62]

Demon pullers, more than any other cleric–healers of proven medical–magical knowledge, identified themselves openly with the possession of 'abominable skills' and actively sought to pass their knowledge on to their students. This was particularly so during the

Imperial Era when demon pullers were by far freer and numerically greater than they were in earlier periods. So, what practical advantage did students of the healing arts expect to gain from 'communicating' with or 'inheriting' the attributes of Satnael?

The primary advantage was their ability to command a greater body of medical and extramedical knowledge, and to perform a wider range of magical prayers than other cleric–healers.[63] Informants believed that those who befriended Satnael could easily invoke evil spirits, cast a hex and tap the medical–magical knowledge of the spirit world. By contrast, while some informants claimed that certain cleric–healers were able to invoke a few extraterrestrial spirits and make them fulfil their demands[64] without concluding a pact with the Satnael, most informants rejected this claim.

In the end, gaining access to the ostensibly *ne plus ultra* wisdom of the spirit realm must be seen as an advanced intellectual pursuit of a small percentage of medical students.[65] That is why some students of the healing arts who were obsessed with worldly gains were said to be eager to befriend non-benevolent spirits.[66]

As many oral informants asserted, there was a great demand for non-benevolent medicine during the imperial era, particularly among the privileged classes. This demand may have reflected changes that were taking place in the economic and social spheres. Competition in the business sector, endless controversies on urban and rural lands, and the efforts of public offices at all levels of the state structure to gain and hold on to their positions tempted many individuals to seek the magico-medical services of cleric–healers. As a result, a growing number of students sought knowledge of the black arts.

Learning Herbal Medicine or Phytotherapy

Unlike the teaching of magical subjects, which was carried out almost exclusively in and around religious institutions, ethno-botanical studies began with rigorous oral instructions and examination of medical texts in religious establishments, and was followed by practical field instruction. Medical students were expected to study closely and memorise the names and uses of medicinal items (i.e., herbal, animal and mineral origin) often under the supervision of their mentors. Medicinal plants were mostly identified using their Ge'ez nomenclatures.[67]

Students studied and wrote down the names and intended uses of each and every medicinal plant. Rote memorisation of the names and purposes of botanicals was a first stage in developing herbal knowledge. [68] While this level of knowledge could be attained by a well-travelled student, to become a truly well-educated 'ethno-botanist' – the goal of dedicated church-based medical students[69] – required the acquisition of more detailed and nuanced knowledge of the multiple uses, effects and modes of preparation of each plant.

Church-educated literati believed that medicinal herbs[70] had been naturally endowed with 'mysterious healing powers', a vital concept that should be properly communicated to medical students. The maxim ዕፅ ያድን ዕፅ ይገድል (herb cures; herb kills) was a reminder of the need for proper knowledge about herbal drugs and their utilisation. Random utilisation of botanical remedies, regarded as 'a shot in the dark', was a rare phenomenon among well-trained cleric–healers. Not only did they recognise the medicinal uses of different botanicals, they also understood that a single plant could act in multiple ways. Drug plants could have 'healing qualities in the roots, poisoning powers in the fruits or flowers, relieving abilities in the stems or branches'.[71] Given the complexity of the subject, it is not surprising that only a few diligent students were able to grasp in-depth herbal knowledge.

Identifying botanical remedies in their natural habitats – *dagga* (highland), *wayna dagga* (mid-highland) and *qolla* (lowland) (i.e., the three major agro-ecological zones) – was a time-consuming but critical learning experience.[72] For knowing drug plants by name was not enough to distinguish how plants of similar species or appellations could be used.[73] For this reason, teachers needed to take their students to the field to gain hands-on experience of various medicinal plants.[74]

A medical student must also obtain adequate instruction in the rituals and procedures associated with herbal medicaments. For this reason, cleric–healers often expounded the idea that plucking, uprooting and even touching drug plants should be done very carefully. They stressed that plants, like human beings, had been endowed with a 'life force'. Failure to grasp the validity of this principle or to apply the correct method of interacting with drug plants was tantamount to mutual destruction.[75]

In this connection, students of the healing arts were given lessons on how to evade risks and apply the right 'interactive' methods with herbal drugs. The parable: 'If [a] herb is respected, it respects' confirmed the importance of handling medicinal herbs with extreme care, personal cleanliness and ritual purity.[76] In addition, a drug plant could lose its curative virtues should its secret (or Ge'ez) name and its reputed use be disclosed.[77] Broadly speaking, mastering the complex set of highly ritualised rules and procedures for identifying, collecting, preparing and administering drug plants was an important component of the herbal training. Together, these elements ensured that practitioners of herbal medicine maintained a state of ritual purity which was essential for producing effective herbal cures. All of these purportedly indispensable aspects of herbal instructions had to be studied carefully so that a student could attain the required level of proficiency. At the same time, this knowledge needed to be kept secret to protect lay people from the deleterious effects of self-medicating with poisonous or strong herbal drugs.

A richly varied body of written materials related to herbal instruction exists. Some of these date back to the sixteenth century. From these texts, one can identify a number of common lessons cleric–healers taught their disciples on the subject of ritual purity. Cleric–healers placed great emphasis on the importance of cutting or digging out medicinal herbs using specific instruments, such as spears, knives or sharpened wood (often from an olive tree) of particularly shaped handle and handling position. They also stressed the need to approach drug plants with the utmost respect such as by prostrating before them,[78] being naked, cutting one's neck-cord (a piece of thread that served as a badge of Christianity) or reciting some prayers. Students were also taught how and when herbs should be collected, including to use the right or left hand for collecting plants, the importance of standing to the east or west of a plant, and the use of a baby or an old woman or a cat or a dog attached to a herb. They were instructed that some plants needed to be collected under a clear sky, while others were only approached very early in the morning before urinating and without uttering a word, while others were approached at mid-day or mid-night; during five *pagumen*;[79] at new year's day; the first day of a month; or on Tuesdays or

Thursdays. Observing taboos such as sexual continence was also vital for achieving effective results. Likewise, some herbs had to be collected after placing or sprinkling items such as salt, bread, Maria Theresa dollars or birr, milk, honey, linseed, common cress and malt, while others were dug up after scarifying a chicken on the spots where medicinal herbs had been uprooted.[80]

In addition, students needed to master meticulous theoretical and practical instructions for the proper preparation of herbal medicines. These included learning whether a medicinal plant should be prepared fresh, or crushed, dried, pulverised, buried, soaked in water, heated, roasted or boiled. Pounding botanicals using a new wooden or stone mortar, boiling them in a new cooking pot singly or together with some beans or chicken broth and filtering them was important in order to extract the required 'dose' without being contaminated or losing their 'potency,' 'taste' or 'flavour'.[81] Learning how to control strong medicines with antidotes such as whey, butter milk, yoghurt, coffee, linseed or lemon juice was another area of medical training. In addition, knowing the intrinsic nature and after effects of drug plants and how to administer antidotes against strong medicines was a critical quality for a properly trained student. The inclusion of honey and butter[82] in the preparation of most herbal drugs appeared to have similar importance.

Measuring and administering medicaments were two important aspects of learning herbal medicine.[83] Though absolute measurements were totally unknown, cleric–healers always taught their students how to use relative measurements in the preparation of herbal medicaments, such as different-sized spoons (made of horn) for powdered medicines; finger-joint lengths or digits for uncrushed medicinal roots or barks; and cups and drinking glasses of various sizes (made of clay or horn)[84] for herbal concoctions or extractions. They also instructed their disciples in the techniques of plastering, poulticing, gargling, washing the whole or the affected body with herbal concoctions, chewing or sucking medicinal roots or barks, snuffing or instilling medicinal drops, and licking the ashes of burnt herbs. Cleric–healers always emphasised the idea that drug plants would be more effective if administered using the right measuring techniques and in accordance with the age, medical history and the nature of their patients' sickness.[85]

Cleric–healers also taught their students how to classify herbal medicines as 'hot–cold' and how to use 'hot' medicines for 'cold' illnesses and vice versa. The concept of hot–cold was largely based on the idea of differentiating herbal remedies by using olfactory or gustatory senses. By using this method, a medical student should be able to distinguish the right medicinal plant from other plants with similar structures or appearance.

The therapeutic principle of hot–cold, commonly referred to as *contraria contraries*, appears to have been a legacy of ancient Greco–Arab medical thought. This ancient medical idea, arising largely from the theory of the four cardinal humours, permeated Ethiopian medical tradition. Strelcyn compared three local Ethiopian manuscripts with three other Ethiopian texts 'which had lain down in the British Museum for over a century'.[86] He found remarkable similarities between all these texts and 'the third and fourth books of Avicenna's *Canon of Medicine*'.[87] It remains unclear how many cleric–healers had access to Galenic treatises. However, it would appear that many of the herbal and dietetic prescriptions employed by cleric–healers were influenced by Galenic medical texts which are known to have circulated in Ethiopia.[88] Cleric–healers offered their students lessons on the imbalance of the four biological fluids, and their corresponding dietetic and medicinal treatments, albeit in a fragmentary and mechanical fashion.[89]

The idea of humoural imbalance was an important medical concept in classifying and conceptualising the aetiology of certain illnesses and their corresponding cures.[90] These imbalances were treated with the help of drugs classified crudely as being emetics, laxatives, cathartics, narcotics, astringents, expectorants and so on, with or without special diets and other therapeutic procedures such as cupping or blood-letting. At the same time, it is important to note that indigenous definitions of sickness and health went beyond the imbalance of the bodily fluid. Good health also required striking a state of equilibrium with physiological, spiritual, cosmological, ecological and social forces.[91]

The complex procedures involved in gathering, processing and administering various botanical medications, described above, explain why the acquisition of a limited amount of theoretical instruction, along with the ability to memorise the names and attributes of medicinal plants, could not enable a medical student to master herbal medicine. It also indicates why, in the end, only a limited number of medical students could gain access to the whole edifice of verbal and practical instructions on herbal remedies, and why healers who possessed this knowledge were so highly regarded. At the same time, the failure of some students to achieve this high level of expertise did not necessarily prevent them from practising herbal medicine. Thus the quality of herbal medicine that was practised varied. This truth points to an important fact that there was no formal accreditation process, or definitive set of examinations that a student needed to pass in order to claim to be a well-trained cleric–healer.

A point that merits mention is how much the ecology of the Amhara region was suited to learning the herbal lore during the 1920s and 1930s. As many informants noted, with some degree of nostalgia, the forest cover during this time was so vast that they had no problem obtaining curative herbs from nature's 'pharmaceutical industry'.[92] This meant that cleric–healers did not always need to travel to remote places to instruct their students or in search of medicinal plants.[93] This situation changed following the Italian occupation. Forest regulations, which had begun under Menelik, ceased to be enforced until the passage of new regulations in the 1960s. Loss of forest during this interim period made it more difficult for healers to locate herbal medicines and to instruct their students.

Conclusion

The quality of medico-magical trainings enabled medical students to have specialised knowledge that ensured their privileged position in the medical marketplace. Cleric–healers' mastery of Ge'ez and the art of writing[94] were powerful tools for co-opting and maintaining ultimate control over healing practices. They translated all the medical information they obtained from non-cleric and preliterate healers into Ge'ez, a body of knowledge inaccessible to non-church-based healers;[95] in other words, the body of medical knowledge generated by non-cleric–healers was, over time, incorporated, preserved and transmitted within the framework of the church-based medical system. This gave cleric–healers a clear competitive advantage over non-cleric–healers, and it contributed to their reputation as healers who possessed highly privileged sets of skills and knowledge.[96]

Figure 8: A magical prayer against the devil

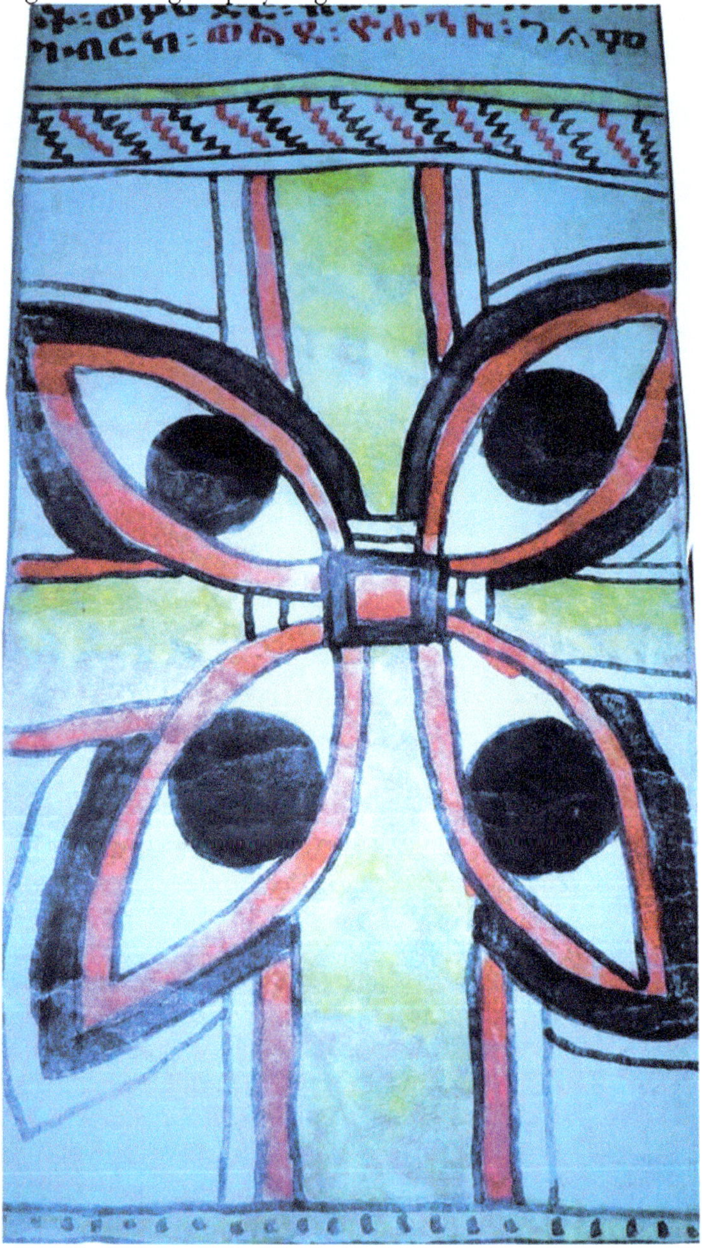

Source: IES Ms. No. 666

Figure 9: A personal protective amulet

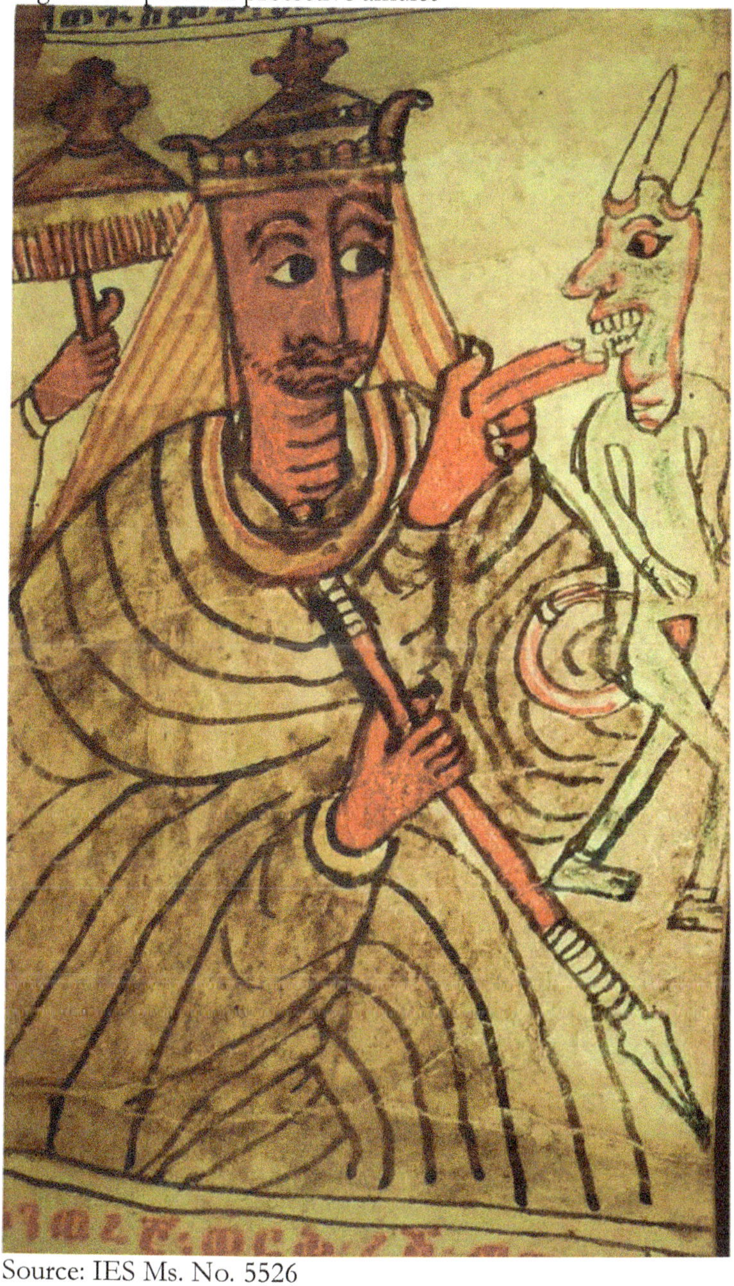

Source: IES Ms. No. 5526

1 Oral informants nos. 4, 11, 12, 18, 20, 21, 36, 39 and 59.

2 The traditional Ethiopian staple food was made mostly of teff (*Erogrostis tef*) or *gabse* (*Hordeum valgare*).

3 Kidane Mariam Getahun, *Traditional Ethiopian Student* (Amharic) (Addis Ababa: Tensae Zagubae Printing Press, 1954, E.C.).

4 Oral informants nos. 2, 27, 30 and 35.

5 Since the early days of the introduction of Christianity into Ethiopia in the fourth century CE, many religious texts originating from Greek, Egypt, Syria and Jerusalem had been translated into Ge'ez. Translations of foreign literary sources, including those of Arabic texts, and other original works were said to have been accomplished between the fourteenth and the seventeenth centuries, a period of Ethiopian history known commonly as 'the golden age of Ge'ez literature'. Since the fourteenth century, texts on Ethiopian sacred figures have begun to be produced.

6 See *Lefafe Tsediq* (*The Bandlet of Righteousness* or *Book of the Dead*) and *Arde'et* (*The Magic of the Disciples*).

7 Wallis Budge, *The Book of the Saints of the Ethiopian Church*, 4 volumes (Cambridge: Cambridge University Press, 1928). For a bibliography on *malk*, see J. Simon, 'Bibliography on Malkee', *Orientalia*, 10 (1941): 307–308; and for a comprehensive list of hagiographical works, see Knife-Rigb Zelleke, 'Bibliography of Ethiopic Hagiographical Traditions', *JES*, 13(2) (1975): 57–102; for a description of the sacred objects of the church, see Marcel Griaule, 'Les règles de l'eglise', *Journal Asiatique*, 221 (1932): 1–41. A good example of this is a prayer text called *Hasura Masqal* (Rampart of the Cross).

8 IES, MSS nos. 330, 792, 2378 and 939.

9 Deborah Lifchitz, *Textes ethiopien magico-religieux* (Paris. L'Institut d'ethnologie, 1940), 15. The book constitutes the facsimiles and translations of a number of magico-religious texts.

10 Sylvain Grebaut, 'L' hymne: invocation Lesana Sab'e', *Aethiopica*, 1 (1935): IES, MS nos. 146 and 463.

11 Sylvain Grebaut, 'Le prière Sayfa Malakot', *Aethiopica*, 1 (1936).

12 Deborah Lifchitz, *Textes ethiopien magico-religieux*, 13.

13 These are some of the common titles given to a compendium of permissible magico-religious prayers. See, for example, IES, MS no. 3000.

14 See, for example, Sylvain Grebaut, 'Noms ésotériques de Dieu rêvéles aux archanges', *Aethiopica*, 4 (1934). Several magical prayers containing the secret names of Christ were composed in the name of Solomon, Moses, Saint Endrias, the Disciples, Enoch, Saint Thomas, Abraham,

David, Simeon, Sirak, Saint Cyprien, Mary and the Archangels. See Stefan Strelcyn, 'La magie ethiopienne,' 150–151.

15 A passage from this text reads, 'Everybody who believes, and reads, by these [secret] names of Christ let him be saved from sin and from all bad and wicked and treacherous man [sic], and from all disease[s] of soul and body, and from all demons and evil spirits . . . and he shall be like the 12 Disciples.' See Enno Littmann, 'Arde'et: The Magic Book of the Disciples', *JAOS* XXV, (1904): 26. See also Rene Basset, *Enseignement de Jesus-Christ a ses disciples et prieres magiques* (Paris: Librairie de L'Art Independent, 1896).

16 Prayer texts such as መልክአ ውቃቢ (Image of Guardian Spirits) and መስሀብ መላእክት ወመስሀበ ቅዱሳን ወባሕታውያን (Prayers to Invoke Angels, Saints and Hermit Monks) were more than ordinarily permissible prayers that were recited to come into contact with, and conjure up, benevolent spirits. The majority of the clergy had difficulty accessing this group of prayers, while hermit monks were said to be the principal repositories. See IES, MSS nos. 495, 1020 and 2199. A similar prayer is also found in MS no. 2417(B).

17 Inside the many personal amulets and charms (with or without images or figures, and in scroll, accordion or book forms), one finds names of people (mostly of baptismal ones to whom these prayers were copied) being inserted in various places so as to help them attain their immediate or long-term objectives. See for, example, IES, MSS nos. 144, 145, 147, 148, 151, 155–159, 163–172, 178, 179, 181, 186, 190–192, 195, 217–221, 224–239, 403–416, 437, 445–456, 458–459, 473–491, 498, 500–674, 680, 698, 1998 and 2976.

18 Written sources do not agree on the production dates of these materials; the time gap is huge, falling between the fourteenth and seventeenth centuries. For a related discussion, see Gezahegn Getachew, 'The Various Characters of Hagiographies' (Amharic) *Proceedings of the Workshop on the Ethiopian Church Yesterday, Today and Tomorrow* Addis Ababa, 18–19 April 2002, 90–114.

19 Sprinkling a patient with holy water and massaging his or her body with a cross for a week or more has been the most dominant curative method of the church. Several monasteries and churches, such as Debra Libanos, Zeqwala, Shenkora and Mitaq, to mention only a few, have been known for their therapeutically powerful *tabal.*

20 An ecclesiastic who commanded a good deal of magico-religious knowledge enjoyed a very high degree of acceptance and admiration. Oral informants nos. 18, 20, 30 and 42.

21 Oral informant no. 38.

22 *Awda Nagast* is the only printed text in which a few non-permissible magico-religious prayers were made available for the first time: prayers to obtain the love of the opposite sex or other human beings, respect, appointment, money, wealth and to maintain one's position; prayers against the enemy and a magical attack from the *tila wagi* (an act of murder by piercing the shadow of a person); prayers to undo magic spells; prayers for binding and defeating demons (or Solomon's Net); prayer to render an enemy inactive or indolent; prayer to protect a person from anything injurious; prayers to unravel the secrets of others and to have visions, dreams or revelations. See *Awda Nagast* (1953 E.C.), 148–174.

23 Oral informants nos. 4, 35, 37 and 57. For a variety of magico-medical prayers, see Sylvain Grebaut, *Recueil de texts magiques ethiopiens* (Paris, Librairie orientaliste Paul Geuthner, 1939).

24 One may also presume that magico-religious prayers being recited without their *gabir* may not attain their intended results or they may not be as important as they ought to be.

25 Mekonnen Bishaw, 'Integrating Indigenous and Cosmopolitan Medicine in Ethiopia', unpublished PhD dissertation (Southern Illinois University, 1988), 60.

26 Jean Doresse, *Ethiopia: Ancient Cities and Temples* (London: Elek Books, 1959), 121.

27 'Whoever is found in possession of magical prayers . . . shall be punished like an idolater, and his property shall be given to the Church,' stated one of the texts written by the Emperor. More common 'was the use of magical prayers by members of the Christian community, including the clergy'; a crime that was punishable 'on pain of death'. See Tadesse Tamrat, *Church and State in Ethiopia 1270–1527* (Oxford: The Clarendon Press, 1972), 235.

28 Oral informants nos. 40, 41, 42 and 43; Reidulf K. Molvaer, 'Medical Anthropology Topics of Relevance for Health Workers and Students of Health in Ethiopia' (Addis Ababa: UNICEF/Ministry of Health, 1987), 94.

29 To obtain copies of religious texts, students lacking both the skill and the necessary resources had to serve their teachers for a long time until they acquired the requisite copying skill and permission to copy teachers' texts. See Tekle Tsadik Mekuria, *History of Ethiopia: From Emperor Lebne Dengel to Emperor Tewodros* (Amharic) (Addis Ababa: Tensae Zagubae Printing Press, 1953, E.C.), 9.

30 But this momentary achievement that contradicted the envisaged aims and purposes of church-based medicine might render a student's final success undeserving (Oral informant, no. 20).

31 Oral informant, no. 2. Adopting made-up names was one of the oldest traditions of religious students; especially those who decided to become a hermit monk did not reveal their true identities to their colleagues or their whereabouts to their families.

32 Ibid.

33 The refusal to live within the limitations imposed upon them was an anticipated reaction of students who had been beleaguered by 'unfulfilled desire, exhausted patience, endless frustration and distressfulness', noted an informant (Oral informant, no. 21).

34 The informant alleged that it was with a magic spell called XGr mLS (a magic prayer to bring a person back to his master) that the student was destined to return and avail himself to his teacher.

35 Ibid. Another student who was caught red-handed while stealing a drug under preparation for the teacher's son was thrown out from a school without probation and went to another teacher.

36 Oral informants nos. 11 and 19.

37 Taddele Gadlie, *Qene and Qene Games to Cherish the Past* (Amharic), 2nd edition. (Addis Ababa: Gutenberg Printing Press, 1997, E.C.), 12.

38 Oral informants nos. 2, 21, 35 and 37: they argued that it was a deliberate strategy of experienced cleric–healers to deter their students from venturing into unwarranted experiments and facing risky outcomes.

39 For a correlation of words and numbers, see Habte Mariam Workneh, *Traditional Ethiopian Curriculum* (Amharic) (Addis Ababa: Berhanena Selam Printing Press, 1962, E.C.), 238.

40 Oral informants nos. 2, 19, 20, 22, 30, 31, 35 and 37. A very good example of this has been the placement of instructions on how to apply Satnael's prayers on an entirely separate page(s). See MS no. 2417 (D), 1–4; 82–83.

41 For a few cases of this writing technique, see IES, MSS nos. 2417(C), 84 and 2417(I), 32.

42 Oral informant, no. 2: the same informant attributed *nagara dabtara* to eight prominent cleric–healers, whom he referred to as 'four-eyed' (or highly educated) scholars, teaching in Gojjam and Gondar around the middle of the twentieth century. Based on the ages of these elderly Orthodox savants, the relative date of this 'invention' at the latest may have been in the early twentieth century. However, this assertion is hardly acceptable, for there have been ample tip-offs on the application of similar writing techniques in quite a number of manuscripts from previous periods. Temesgen dubs this writing technique *nagara woyra* (something that resembles olive), Temesgen Gebre, *Autobiography*, 30.

43 Along with Ge'ez, Amharic was frequently employed to write fragments of prescriptions and/or instructions at the bottom of magico-religious and magico-medical prayers.

44 Oral informant, no. 11.

45 Oral informant, no. 19.

46 Ibid.

47 Jacques Mercier, 'Les dabtara et le vocabulaire de la magie et de la medicine,' *Documents histoire civilisation ethiopienne* RCP 230 (Paris: Centre national de la recherche scientifique, 1976), 117.

48 Oral informants, nos. 20 and 27.

49 *Awda Nagast* (1953, E.C.), 37–38. Albeit with too much personal effort, many non-Mizan Nafas students were allowed to study the black arts (oral informant no. 27).

50 As recruitment was under teachers' jurisdiction, even a Mizan Nafas student, on account of his unwanted conduct, was prevented from learning the healing arts because his teacher branded him 'a potentially dangerous person who would not hesitate to harm others' (oral informant no. 27), and for a similar experience in the 1970s (oral informant no. 28).

51 The following list may demonstrate the variety of evil–magical prayers. Some of them have been adapted from Strelcyn. Provoking discord among relatives, families, neighbours or friends, and inducing dissension and divorce among spouses (መስተጻልዕ) causing serious illness (መስተሐምም), chasing a person away from his place of residence (መስተባርር), turning a person insane or into an idiot (መስተአብድ ዘይስልብ ልበ ሰብእ), killing a person or an opponent (መቅተል መቅተለ ፀር), causing sexual impotency (መቅተል ዘእስኪት) making a woman childless or infertile (ዘእያመክን ብእሲት) making a person dumb or blind (ማዕሰረ ልሳን ሰውር ዘአይንት) and so on, have been some of the most common titles of evil–magical spells. See Stefan Strelcyn, 'La magie ethiopienne', p. 154. Others included invoking terrestrial and extraterrestrial spirits for magical purposes. To conjure the spirits of the air, the Zar, demons and other lesser spirits (ለምስሀብ ዘአየር ምስሀበ ዛር ምስሀበ አጋንንት ምስሀበ ሸይጣን የወረን ማቅረቢያ), for magically stealing the property of others (መስለቢያ), for spoiling home-brewed alcoholic drinks (ለጠጅ ለጠላ ማጥፊያ ወይም ማበላሻ), to be able to see evil demons (አጋንንት ለማየት), for sending destructive rain or hail (ለበረድ ለዝናብ), to bring and keep a woman without her will (አምፅአ ብእሲት ምስሀበ እንስት ለማዕሰረ ብእሲት), to torture a person by sending stones or filthy substances (ለአንደርብ ሙራደ እብን), to make a person flatulent (የፈስ አስማተ ፈስ), to make a person's wealth and business unproductive (መድፍነ ሐብት ወገቢያ), exposing one's enemy to the entering of an evil spirit (ጠላትህን ጋኔን ለማስመታት making a person

indolent or inactive (አስማተ መፍዝዝ ወመቅዝዝ አስማተ መፍዝዝ ወመደንግዝ, have been additional titles of evil magic spells.

52 Though there have been several types of inherently evil or non-permissible magical prayers, the following ones may be taken as examples of 'helpful' or 'non-malevolent' prayers: to attain economic improvement (ለመንድግ), for blessing one's property (ለበረከት), to attract money and prosperity (ምስሀበ ንዋይ መፍትሔ ሐብት), to succeed in business and attract clients (ለገበያ)), to prevent cattle from dying (ከብት ለሚሞትበት), to protect one from thieves and brigands (ለሌባ ወቀማኛ), against the magical influence of the *Salabi* (ለእርኝ ለወተት ለጠላ ወለጠጅ ሰላቢ) to protect one from and defeat one's opponent (የጠላት ለፀር ጠላት በተነሳብህ ጊዜ መድፊነ ፀር), to get respect (ግርማ ሞገስ), to help in a court case or litigation (ለሙግት ሙግት ወክርክር), to help a person become a speedy writer, have a good memory, to learn and retain religious lessons, to have good magical wisdom and skill (በአንተ መክሥተ ትምህርት ወአፍጥነ ድርሰት ለአፅንዖ ትምህርት ለአፅንዖ ቃለ እግዚአብሔር አስማተ ጥበብ አስማተ ሥርወ ለጥበብ መፍትሔ ዕደ ጥበበ), to be a good academician and calligrapher or copyist (ለቀለም ለፅህፈት), to understand the contents of books (መክሰተ ሚስጥረ መጻሕፍት ወድርሰት), to play the harp (ለበገና), to know or to unravel the secrets of others (በእንተ መክሰተ ሚስጥር), to have a dream or vision (ለራእይ ለሕልም መክሠተ ሕልም), to induce or experience sound sleep (ለእንቅልፍ), to create illusion (ለምትሐት), to fly in the air (ለምህዋረ ሠረገላ), to escape from prison (የእግር ብረት መስበሪያ ለእስራት), against fire (ለእሳት), against hail or thunder bolts (ለበረድ ለሙብረቅ ጸሎተ በረድ), against locusts (ለአንበጣ), against porcupine, monkeys and apes (ለጃርት ለጦጣም ለዝንጀሮም), to protect domestic animals from predators (መስተሐድር), to help a woman find a husband (ልጃገረድ ባል እንድታገባ), to be loved by the opposite sex (ለፍቅር ለመውደድ አስማተ ፍቅር ሴትን ወንድ እንዲወድ መስተፋቅር), for the fidelity of one's spouse (ዐቃቢ ሕግ ለሕገ ጠብቅ), to protect a wife from being abused by her husband (ሴትን ባልዋ እንዳይመታት), a solution for a jealous woman (ሴት ስትቀና), to make a slave or servant faithful to his or her master (ለማዕሠረ ገብር ለባሪያ ማዕሠር), against (or to postpone) death (ማዕሰረ ሞት), to keep cats from escaping (ማዕሰረ ድመት), to bring a woman back to her husband or a domestic slave or a servant to his master (እግረ ድመት)), a cure for a crying baby (ለሚአለቅስ ልጅ) against bed-wetting (ሌሊት ለሚሸና), to bring rain (ለዝናም), to make oneself invincible (ለመሰዉር), against intoxication (ለስካር), to help a person become orator or articulate (ዘያስተናግር), to disband a conspiracy (ነገረ በትን), against bullets, swords and sticks (ለጥይት ለቅንአት ለበትር), to fight against the magical medicine of seers and magicians (ለአቃቤ ሥራይ), and a prayer to overcome fear (ለፍርሀት), and so on.

53 Siegbert Ulzig (ed.), *Encyclopaedica Aethiopica*, 640.

54 This huge manuscript, compiled under the sponsorship of Jacques Mercier in the 1970s, was copied from the personal collection of more than a dozen cleric–healers. All these prayers were copied on paper (most probably by the same cleric–healers) and transferred to a British millionaire by the name of Sanfogg who, in turn, donated them to the Institute of Ethiopian Studies in the early 1990s. It is not clear how the scribes whose names have been indicated at the beginning of many of the magic prayers made the deal with the French ethnologist to whom they revealed and copied their personal medico-magical materials during the Darg regime. However, the presence of several magical prayers under similar titles also demonstrated the difference in size, content and manner of application of church-affiliated medicine and healing and the various methods through which cleric–healers collected their manuscripts.

55 Allan Young, 'Magic as a Quasi-Profession: The Organization of Magic and Magical Healing Among the Amhara', *Ethnology* 14(3) (1975): 255.

56 Isaiah 14:12.

57 For a description of different demons and their area of expertise, see Enoch 19:10–29.

58 *Mawares* would mean literally 'acquisition or adoption by a human being of the wisdom, attributes and assistances of the leader of evil spirits, Satnael and his minions'.

59 Allan Young, 'The Practical Logic of Amhara Traditional Medicine' In *African Therapeutic Systems*, edited by Z. A. Ademumagun, et al. (Los Angeles: Crossroads Press, 1979), 84.

60 For different versions of Satnael's prayers and those of the items recommended in the ritual, see MSS nos. 386 Part III (not paginated); 2417 (C), 131–139; 2417 (D) 1–4, 76–79; Stefan Strelcyn, *La magie ethiopienne*, 155–157.

61 IES, MS no. 2417 (C), 142.

62 Oral informant, no. 17.

63 It is stated in the instruction that with the use of this powerful prayer a person could supposedly perform more than 40 extraordinary magical activities.

64 Though he did not mention their educational background, Weissleder came across an outlaw and a judge 'who are definitely known to possess . . . powers' of using the spirit of darkness'. See Weissleder, 'The Political Ecology', 78.

65 Some religious figures were known to have gone through the rituals of 'inheritance' to create mystical relationships with the saints, angels and other sacred figures of the church. The course of action for creating friendship with holy figures was said to be an extremely rigorous and

daunting task that a pious person, such as a celibate monk or an anchorite interested in doing so, had to fast and pray in the strictest solitude for not less than four years. A person after 'inheritance' would assume extraordinary virtues in communicating with, and getting the assistance of, sacred figures so as to help the sick, foresee the future and other similar beneficent deeds (Oral informants, nos. 21 and 32). A number of stories have been recounted about the *gadl* (or miracles) of several monastic holy figures known to have commanded and served the devil. See, for instance, *Gadla Takla Haymanot*, Chapter 48; for a similar assertion, see *Tamra Mariam* (Miracles of Mary). This shows that to draw a clear-cut boundary between a purely religious and magical method of commanding evil spirits is not simple.

66 According to the church, many people fell into the snare of Satan because they did not know that Satan had an exceptional power of exploiting their weaknesses, such as presenting to them very attractive worldly ideas and seducing them into committing sins and, ultimately, detaching them from God.

67 Amharic had been utilised as a spoken language at least since the thirteenth century, and it became a written language replacing Ge'ez only during the reign of Emperor Tewedros (1855–1868).

68 The names of plants occurred in a wide range of local languages, as well as in Arabic. Lexical examination of sixteenth-century written sources enabled Strelcyn to differentiate about 175 Ethiopian plants bearing Arabic names, see Stefan Strelcyn, 'Les chapitres concernant les plantes d'un lexique Arabe-Ethiopien du XVIs', *Roczn. Orient*, XXXI (1968).

69 Not to do so was a source of confusion: to utilise correctly drug plants identified by the same name(s) when these names may have been used for identifying different medicinal plants.

70 Cleric–healers firmly believed that application of herbal medicines had a mythical origin, going back to the time of King Solomon to whom God had shown the medicinal importance of about 550 herbs, including honey, butter and milk. According to this mythical belief, which provided cleric–healers a certain degree of legitimacy to their vocation, it was at the insistence of Solomon that the Creator of the Universe agreed to teach him the secrets of herbal medicines. See IES, MS no. 2444. Messing, recording a localised version of a similar mythology, says that 'God gave 1 000 special "medicines" to Jesus on Christmas (a sort of birthday gift) and that Jesus and the angels taught these "medicines" to the *member* [a cleric–healer].' See Simon Messing, 'The Highland Plateau Amhara of Ethiopia', unpublished PhD dissertation (University of Pennsylvania, 1957), 672.

71 Alemayehu Moges, 'Traditional Ethiopian Medicine,' 111.

72 Oral informants nos. 4 and 18. They also underlined the importance of differentiating correctly between parasitic (epiphytes), monoscious (single sex) and dioscious (bisexual) plants. The same is also true for multi-purpose herbs commonly known as *hulagab*, which could be used singly or in combination with other medicinal plants.

73 Dawit and Ahadu have cited about 17 vernacular names of drug plants representing two or more plant species; see Dawit Abebe and Ahadu Ayehu, *Medicinal Plants and Enigmatic Health Practices of Northern Ethiopia* (Addis Ababa: Berhanena Salam Printing Press, 1993), 24–25.

74 Oral informants nos. 1, 2, 11, 19, 32 and 57.

75 Oral informants nos. 11, 22, 24, 27 and 30.

76 See Alemayehu Moges, 'Traditional Ethiopian Medicine,' *8th International Conference of Ethiopian Studies*, Addis Ababa, I (1984), 133.

77 It was to build unbounded trust in their healing power more than maintaining the efficacy of the medicinal substances that cleric–healers did not want to disclose the names of medicinal plants to others. Since most herbal medical texts have been fraught with these seemingly unintelligible instructions and their alleged utilisation, they could be interesting aspects of future ethno-botanical investigation from which a great deal of the secret of herbal medicine could be unravelled.

78 This procedure was particularly vital while collecting 'powerful' medicinal herbs.

79 The thirteenth month (or leap year) on the Ethiopian calendar. Oral informants nos. 1, 2, 11, 19, 32 and 57.

80 Oral informants nos. 4, 18, 22 and 30.

81 Oral informants nos. 4 and 30.

82 The medicinal quality of honey and butter has been a highly exaggerated notion.

83 Oral informants nos. 1, 2 and 57. Well-trained cleric–healers being attentive to the most common allegations against indigenous medicine, such as lack of 'appropriate dosage' and utilisation of 'sham' herbal drugs, defended themselves, saying that such charges were totally unheard of during the early twentieth century. In those days there were no leanings to this kind of unacceptable venture, argued informants, because medical students were subjected to rigorous ethical and medical trainings.

84 In the post-Italian period these locally made writing utensils had been gradually replaced with factory-produced items.

85 Oral informants nos. 4, 22 and 30.

86 Stefan Strelcyn, 'Ethiopian Medical Treatises as a Source for the Study of Early Amharic', trans. C. C. Patterson and A. K. Irvine, *International Congress of Africanists* (n.d.), 107. After studying a cleric's medical text

from Begemdir, Strelcyn remarked that Ethiopian medical texts, extracted or abridged from larger foreign treatises, were specially tailored to deal with local maladies and to adapt to local situations. Stefan Strelcyn, 'Les medecines du Begamder et du Tchelga (Ethiopie) D'Abba Garred', *Africana Bulletin* 5 (1966): 53–54.

87 Quoted in Allan Young, 'Medical Beliefs and Practices of Begemder Amhara', unpublished PhD dissertation (University of Pennsylvania, 1970), 174.

88 Institute of Ethiopian Studies, MS no. 992; Haddis Gebre Meskel, *Book of Medicine: Traditional Ethiopian Medicine* (Amharic) (London: Haddis Publications, 1988), 145–147; Ahadu Ayehu, 'Book of Herbs,' 9–16; Strelcyn examined ancient Ethiopian manuscripts containing dietetic and therapeutic ideas of the Greco–Arab world. See Stefan Strelcyn, 'Les ecrits medicaux ethiopiens', *JES*, 3(1) (1965): 82–103; Stefan Strelcyn, *Medecine et plantes d'Ethiopie: les traites medicaux ethiopiens*, 115–148. As Young put it plainly, 'Galenic treatises have circulated in Christian Ethiopia; but they are known to very few cleric healers and have had no persuasive effect on cleric healers' understanding of health and sickness.' Allan Young, 'Internalizing and Externalizing Medical Belief Systems: An Ethiopian Example', *Social Science and Medicine*, 10(3/4) (1976): 155.

89 An informant, explaining the application metaphorically without understanding this medical idea, said, 'Most cleric healers would simply apply this medical idea in a manner similar to operating a TV set even if They did not have the slightest knowledge how the equipment was manufactured' (Oral informant no. 1).

90 Humoral imbalance was conceived as a disorder that would make a person (depending on the type of humour he was born with) vulnerable to specific illness(es): a bilious person was said to be mostly attacked with severe headache, tumour, jaundice, leprosy and mental diseases; a sanguine with eye diseases, measles, and boils; a phlegmatic with vitiligo and partial paralysis; while a melancholic was known to be vulnerable to body sores such as scabies and the like. See Stefan Strelcyn, *Médecine et plantes D'Ethiopie: les traites medicaux ethiopiens*. 116–148, 156–166.

91 Norbert Vecchiato, 'Traditional Medicine', in *The Ecology of Health and Disease in Ethiopia*, edited by Helmut Kloos and Zein Ahmed Zein (Colorado: Westview Press, 1993), 157–159.

92 Informants also reiterated that during this period the degree of forest clearing – either for fuel wood, grazing lands and agronomic practice, including commercial agriculture and human settlement – was not a formidable threat to the plant life and the natural environment.

93 It was during Menelik's reign that the Ministry of Agriculture, entrusted with the huge responsibility of protecting the environment, was

established in the first decade of the twentieth century. One of the ministry's responsibilities was to encourage 'tree planting', reward those 'who planted many trees' and to prohibit the 'indiscriminate felling of trees and the protection of all forests'. See Dessalegn Rahmato, 'Environmentalism and Conservation in Wallo Before the Revolution', *JES*, 31(1) (1998): 59–60.

94 The two religious establishments that were officially authorised to teach especially designed writing lessons or calligraphy (or ya*qum tsehefet*) were Andabet and Afarewanat in Begemdir.

95 Being adept in the art of writing, cleric–healers lost no time in integrating the oral information they obtained from secular healers into their medical handbooks. This suggests that cleric–healers were in the habit of recording newly discovered medicinal plants or herbs. It was most probably after the 1918 influenza epidemic that *bahr zaf* (*Eucalyptus globulus*), a plant introduced to Ethiopia from Australia in the early twentieth century, began to be mentioned in the medical texts of the twentieth century. For a brief remark on the medicinal use and relative efficacy of *bahr zaf* during this epidemic, see Imru Haile Selassie, *From What I Heard and Remember* (Amharic) (Addis Ababa: Addis Ababa University Press, 2001, E.C.), 89.

96 Though questionable, the growth in literacy rate, and the proliferation of writing tools and printing technology in the post-Italian period gave non-cleric healers access to a body of knowledge that was hidden from them and an edge in competition with church-educated healers.

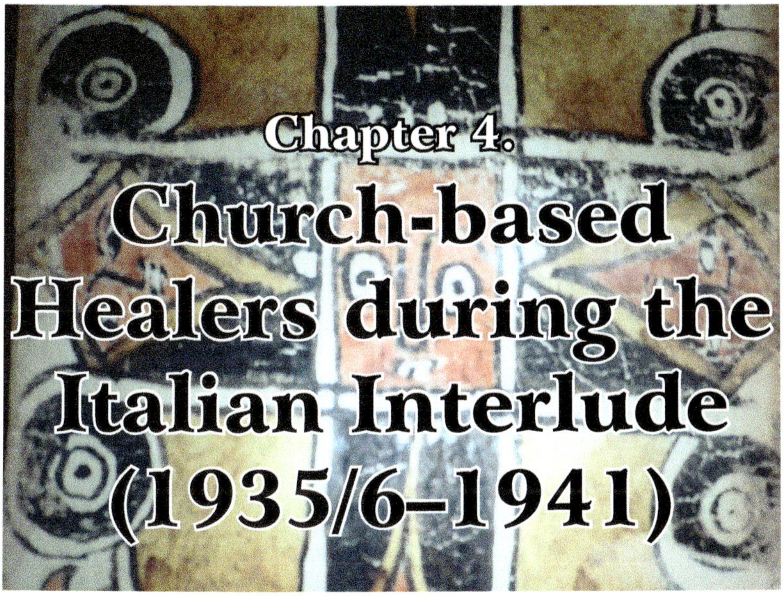

Chapter 4. Church-based Healers during the Italian Interlude (1935/6–1941)

During the early twentieth century church-educated healers served as healthcare providers of indigenous medicine and dominated the medical landscape of Ethiopia. They maintained this position through tight control over esoteric forms of medical knowledge based on their learning of church education. Religious students developed an interest in and joined selected religious institutions to learn church-based medicine. At the same time, Western medicine was able to make only limited advances. However, the dominance of cleric–healers began to weaken, following the Italian occupation in the mid-1930s.

The Italians transformed the medical marketplace in two major ways: (1) by increasing Western medical services, and (2) by attacking Ethiopian religious institutions and church-based healers. As part of their attack, the Italians killed several cleric and non-cleric indigenous healers. This chapter examines the Italian colonial policy towards the Ethiopian Orthodox Tewahedo Church and church-based healers, and why the colonial officials wanted to eliminate them from the scene. It also touches on how the Italians succeeded in beginning to popularise European biomedicine in Ethiopia. Ultimately, it casts a ray of light on how religious institutions endeavoured to maintain church-based medical education and practice in the face of these attacks.

The Italian Health Policy

With the establishment of the Italian administration, though fleeting, the impact of Western medicine began to be felt in Ethiopia. The Italians introduced a large number of Western medical practitioners, primarily to provide medical services to the Italians who accompanied the occupation. The Italians also provided the Ethiopian population with separate medical services. In doing so, they pursued a policy, common in most European colonies, of limiting the costs of medical care; for example, during a typhus outbreak in 1936 only the white population in Addis Ababa initially received the newly developed Weigl vaccine.[1] The seriousness of the situation, however, compelled the Italians to extend Weigl vaccine to the people of Shewa, the provincial centre of the colonial administration. Coinciding with this, the Italians chose to vaccinate local African populations with live smallpox vaccine, rather than bear the cost of importing the safer and more effective vaccine made of the vaccinia virus.[2]

Italian investments in the health of Ethiopians were also selective, targeting diseases that threatened the political and economic interests of the colony; for example, the Italians established provisional hospitals for the native soldiers who were needed to maintain the colonial order. They also established a number of temporary clinics and dispensaries to serve the health needs of the large army of road workers upon whom the Italians depended to create and maintain communications in their colony. Finally, they created *borcelle* (clinics) in many towns for the treatment of venereal diseases among prostitutes and in the brothels in order to protect their workers and soldiers from infection.[3] More general health services were limited to controlling diseases that might spill over into the European population; these included malaria laboratories, eye clinics and anti-epidemic units.

Despite these limitations, the presence in Ethiopia of a large body of Italian health personnel and the increased efficacy of biomedical treatment increased peoples' confidence in the qualitatively distinct mode of Western medicine. By the time of the

Italian invasion, advances in bacteriology and malariology had begun to provide new ways to prevent and treat common diseases. The Italians had played a leading role in carrying out epidemiological studies[4] and initiating effective campaigns against malaria, a disease that was prevalent in Italy at the time. The projects Mussolini launched in Italy for improving the drainage system (as a component of *bonifica integrale*, a comprehensive policy of 'rural upliftment') were part of his anti-malarial public health efforts.[5] The Italians also made efforts to supply the Ethiopian people with limited curative and prophylactic medical services, including disinfection squads, to combat venereal and other transmissible diseases such as smallpox, typhus (particularly louse-borne or epidemic typhus), typhoid-fever and tuberculosis. It should be underlined that the limited 'immunization efforts were launched because Italian medical authorities were afraid that their people would be infected and return to Italy with contagious diseases'.[6]

The Italians observed that 'the native population in the first few months showed itself [sic] mistrustful and did not want to know of our medical cures nor of preventative vaccines against contagious diseases'.[7] The Italian disinfection squads, for example, had difficulty getting accurate information about disease-affected localities in rural areas. Suspicion and lack of trust made the rural public unenthusiastic about co-operating with the squads. However, rural communities had very little real power to stop the mobile teams that periodically administered prophylactic vaccines or fumigated dwellings with disinfectants; for to attempt to do so would result in serious penalties.

Notwithstanding this initial hesitation, the scale of the Italian medical enterprise began to have an effect on Ethiopian attitudes, particularly in urban centres. In addition to Addis Ababa, the capital of Africa Orientale Italiana, in which many healthcare facilities were found, towns such as Harar, Dire Dawa, Gondar, Dessie and Jimma, which served as regional or sub-regional capitals of the colonial administration, received some Western healthcare facilities. In these areas Ethiopians began to appreciate some of the benefits of Western medicine and adopt certain treatment preferences. In contrast to the pre-Italian period, the degree of public acquaintance with the hypodermic needle increased considerably during the occupation; for instance, many Ethiopians appear to have been impressed by the burning sensation and strength-giving calcium preparation administered with a syringe, known popularly as *calcio*. The acclaimed therapeutic value of *calcio* seemed to play a pivotal role in making injectionable treatment acceptable.[8] As occurred elsewhere in Africa, the Ethiopian public soon came to prefer medicine by injection rather than by the swallowing of pills.

By contrast, Ethiopians seem to have had an unbounded fear of surgical procedures.[9] This fear seems to have been related to both Christian and Islamic ideas about the sanctity of the human body. Habte Mariam, an official of the Ethiopian Orthodox Tewahedo Church, explained the public's antipathy towards surgery by quoting an old adage which says: '[N]o one should lose any part of his body after baptism'. Owing to this ingrained belief, a person who had gone through any sort of surgical operation was considered to be a defective or handicapped individual; and any attempt at rectifying the anatomical or physiological problem of the human body with surgical intervention was tantamount to intervening in the flawless creation of God. 'One does not remove a finger which is rotting,'[10] wrote Habte Mariam; and he argued that the dread of losing a part of their body caused people to fear going to a hospital. Owing to this public attitude, the legacy of surgery in the Italian period was not as significant as that of other modes of biomedical practice in Ethiopia.

The Italian administration also pursued a vigorous policy of improving the country's infrastructure – constructing a network of new motor roads, power stations, small industrial firms and healthcare facilities. As a direct result of this effort, a number of permanently based and provisional healthcare facilities were set up. The provision of preventative and curative medical services played a vital role in bolstering Western medical therapies among urban residents and people living around construction sites. Beyond these areas, however, the Italians had little success in expanding Western medical services in rural villages, other than with periodic anti-epidemic campaigns. With the exception of a segment of the population that benefited from Italian medical establishments, the great majority of the Ethiopian public, as in the past, continued to count on the indigenous health practitioners. This is not surprising, given the short duration of Italy's occupation of Ethiopia and the antipathy with which many Ethiopians viewed it.

Italian Attitude Towards Indigenous Healers

Nearly all elderly informants attested to the persistence of indigenous healing practices during the Italian period. This is remarkable, given Italian efforts to suppress these activities. In addition to promoting Western medical treatments, the Italians initiated a full-blown attack on church-educated medical practitioners. These attacks were motivated by several factors. First, the campaign was partly driven by the Italian perception that the church supported Ethiopian resistance to the occupation. Monastic centres suspected of supporting the Ethiopian patriots had a hard time maintaining their integrity and carrying out their activities. The wholesale butchery of the monks of Debre Libanos, a medieval monastery of Saint Tekle Haymanot in Shewa, was ostensibly an act of revenge for their having given shelter to the people who tried to assassinate Graziani, the Italian governor, in Addis Ababa. In the same way, the massacres that took place at Zeqwala, Asabot and numerous other churches and monasteries appear to have been intended to punish the Ethiopian Orthodox Tewahedo Church clergy for sympathising with the patriots.[11]

Although it is unclear to what extent the church actively opposed the Italian occupation, it certainly had reasons for doing so. In an attempt to divide the Ethiopian public, the Italians introduced a policy of alienating the Amhara Ethiopian Orthodox Tewahedo Christians, while favouring non-Amhara, notably the Oromo, and Muslim populations. This policy was based on military and political considerations. The Italians hoped to counterbalance Amhara power by adopting an openly congenial attitude towards the Muslims. By offering official recognition to Islam, the Italians are said to have given enormous financial and moral assistance to Muslims to build new mosques in various towns, including the grand mosque in Addis Ababa and the Shewa Ber mosque in Dessie, and to renovate numerous others, expand Islamic education, and proselytise their religion.[12] This strategy attracted a sizeable number of Muslim Ethiopians to the Italian side.[13]

The Italians further alienated the church by confiscating agricultural lands from Christian landowners and distributing them to Muslim tenants in Wallo. As Sbacchi attested, the net effect of these pro-Muslim policies was to increase anti-colonial sentiment among the Christian public. The Italians had little time to correct the ill-effects of their misguided policy, which was aimed at preventing the Ethiopian Orthodox Tewahedo Christian population from garnering and forging an anti-fascist coalition with their non-Amhara or Muslim compatriots, but which ended in alienating the majority of the Amhara people.[14]

The Ethiopian Orthodox Tewahedo Church became a focus of resistance to the Italian attacks on the Amhara Christian population. An important cause of the church's anti-Fascist sentiment was the Italian destruction of several religious institutions with the aerial bombs poured down by the Regia Aeronautica. This Italian wartime action played a part in positioning the Italians as an enemy of the Ethiopian Orthodox Tewahedo Church. The Italians further alienated the church by attacking religious leaders for refusing to acknowledge their administration. Abuna Petros, the Archbishop of Wollo,[15] for instance, was murdered for repudiating Italian rule and declining to denounce the anti-Fascist fighting forces.[16] With the Abun's assassination, the 'clergy lost confidence in the Italian government',[17] while it reinvigorated the public's resistance against the colonialists.

Accusing the church of rousing and supporting the opposition, the Italians responded by striking out at the clergy, destroying church buildings and monasteries, and looting their treasures.[18] The monasteries and monks were not the only targets of the Italians' efforts to eliminate opposition. They also attacked the small number of Western-educated Ethiopians who had been trained before the occupation.[19] In addition, the Italians directed their attacks against individuals whom they labelled 'seers' and 'soothsayers' (titles associated customarily with lay or hermit monks and cleric–diviners such as church-based healers).[20] The Italian authorities believed that the anti-colonial opposition and patriotic resistance of the Ethiopian public was stimulated by hermit monks, seers and soothsayers whose agitation often focused on the swift end of the occupation and the restoration in jubilation and victory of the Ethiopian crown.[21] The 'shooting of "witch doctors" accused of prophesying the end of fascist rule' has been recorded as one among the many gruesome war crimes of fascist Italy in Ethiopia.[22]

Several *balazar* (spirit medium) spiritual healers, irrespective of their religious faith, were also massacred for allegedly supporting the movement to restore the Ethiopian monarchy. The massacre was described by an eyewitness who narrowly escaped death when several of his *balazar* colleagues were hanged or shot dead at a place called *Holeta* in Shewa. He noted that a powerful *balazar*, a *fitawrari* (commander of the vanguard of a traditional Ethiopian armed force), was among those hanged.[23] This measure seems to have taken place in the wake of the assassination attempt on Graziani. Travelling minstrels accused of transmitting information while playing patriotic songs in taverns and at wedding parties were also executed.[24] In fact, these individuals using their artistic talents played a crucial role in fostering 'a national conscience' and conveying valuable anti-fascist information among the wider public.[25]

The Fascists saw church healers as playing an important role in supporting resistance. They believed that they were providing colonial opponents with magical medicines or prayers to protect them against bullets, thereby boosting the patriots' spirits. In addition, they claimed that the rebels believed that their military victories were aided by a powerful magic spell inscribed by church healers on a black sheep marching in front of their fighting band.[26] They similarly claimed that the day-to-day combat strategy of an important opposition leader in Gojjam was being directed by the advice and recommendations of a cleric–healer. Finally, the resisters, who 'had to rely on traditional doctors and medicine',[27] were believed to have turned to indigenous healers to treat their wounds.

Belief in the role of cleric–healers in the anti-fascist struggle may have pushed the Italians to take ruthless measures against church-educated healers. In the wake of the assassination attempt on governor Graziani, who was believed to have been planning to destroy educational centres of the Ethiopian Orthodox Tewahedo Church and church-educated elites, the Italians launched a campaign of terror against church-based and other healers. It was '[t]o prevent the people from falling under their spell' that Graziani ordered the execution of hermit monks, seers and soothsayers. Between March and July 1937 some 1 500 people were murdered.[28] Hundreds of others were exiled to places such as Denane, Italian Somaliland,[29] 'many of whom never returned'.[30] In addition, 'over 100 deacons and students' of Debra Libanos were put to death at Debra Berhan.[31] The execution of Abuna Petros and the atrocities at Debra Libanos boosted the Ethiopian nationalist consciousness traditionally linked to the Ethiopian Orthodox Tewahedo Church.[32]

Consequences of Resistance

The conditions created by the resistance movement and Italian efforts to suppress it went a long way towards undermining the Italian efforts to control disease and convince the local population of the value of Western medicine. The Italian medical staff was unable to deliver timely medical interventions in vast areas of the countryside occupied by anti-colonial resistance fighters.[33] Combatants were also stricken by epidemics that broke out intermittently.[34] The constant movement of the patriotic bands in rural areas, moreover, facilitated the spread of acute communicable diseases, notably typhus and relapsing fever, in both the fighting units and the civilian population. The instability also gave rise to the dislocation and migration of tens of thousands of the rural people 'to the already overcrowded cities'.[35] Often, these population movements were accompanied by 'acute shortages of food and outbreaks of disease'[36] which, in turn, created fertile ground for endemic diseases to be easily transformed into epidemic outbreaks.

In addition, social dislocations caused by rapid urbanisation encouraged the growth of prostitution, a trade 'initially sponsored by [Italian] officials through the importation of European practitioners'[37] and this, in turn, contributed to a rise in sexually transmitted diseases. The constant movement of the Italian army was also instrumental in encouraging prostitution, and the spread of syphilis and gonorrhoea, which had existed in Ethiopia before the Italian invasion. Cancroid (*karkir*) and *Lymphogranuloms inguinal* (*bambulie* also known as *climatic bubo*), diseases that were evidently introduced into Ethiopia by the Italians,[38] also occurred with considerable frequency.[39]

Furthermore, Leprosy spread during the period of occupation. The Italians rounded up and quarantined stray lepers whom they found in urban areas. Many Ethiopians believed that the Italians killed them. Despite the paucity of first-hand accounts, local oral tradition maintains that in the name of offering feasts, the Italians used to gather and burn many stray lepers alive. Fear of being caught caused many lepers, including those with visible signs of the disease, to flee the cities and seek refuge in the rural areas. The Italian attitude towards leprosy, a disease that manifested itself after a prolonged incubation period, prevented patients with skin and other visible illnesses from seeking treatment from Italian medical establishments. As a matter of fact, the Italians 'forcefully gathered and dumped the sufferers together with other disabled people in the leprosaria', an aide memoire of 'the medieval European leprosaria'.[40] Many of these patients preferred to hide or seek treatment from indigenous healers. This response contributed to the spread of leprosy, skin and other similar diseases in rural areas.[41]

In the face of increased resistance, the Italians recalled Graziani and replaced him with a new Viceroy, the Duke of Aosta, who tried to end the 'execution of suspects on flimsy evidence',[42] and instituted a new policy of conciliation.[43] The Italians continued their attacks on certain religious elements whom they viewed as supporting resistance. However, they were now anxious to make use of the church's influence over the people. They thus attempted to appease the church, proclaiming religious freedom; and not interfering directly in the work of the church, provided that 'there was no occasion to suspect any sympathy with the patriots'.[44] The Duke of Aosta favoured a policy of leaving at liberty church-affiliated and spiritually inspired or possessed individuals. The new viceroy also believed that 'their [the soothsayers'] predictions would be more optimistic if they received government subsidies'.[45] In this he appears to have resurrected a strategy that the Italians had employed before their invasion. According to both oral and written sources, the Italians exploited the mindset of the Ethiopian public by bribing a number of lay and hermit monks to disseminate fabricated prophesies concerning the inevitability of the Italian victory and of the establishment of 'a White Rule' in Ethiopia.[46] In his autobiography, Haile Selassie, writing about these Italian efforts, says: 'During this time, the Italians were busy bringing into play the so-called prophetic words of lay or hermit monks, whom the people recognised as God's messengers, as a major instrument of winning over the uneducated and politically ignorant public.'[47]

The strategy of winning the Ethiopian public through 'spiritually inspired' local agitators, in combination with lavish outpourings of colonial money, had little success in winning over the church. 'Following the reign of terror after the attempt on Graziani's life', no one believed in the 'alleged good intentions of the Duke of Aosta'.[48] Many religious establishments facing a mix of intractable challenges continued to support the patriots in various ways. Most importantly for the history of therapeutics in Ethiopia, the religious institutions that were not destroyed or ransacked by the Fascists succeeded in maintaining their integrity and providing traditional church education during the occupation. In addition, the religious institutions that lay beyond the epicentre of Italian attacks served as safe havens for the numerous clergy fleeing beleaguered or destroyed churches and monasteries. Given the impact of hostilities on health conditions in the country and the disruption of Western medical services, church-based healing and medical education remained very much in demand, and the remaining churches continued to meet these needs.

However, the Italians did succeed in altering the development of church-based healing through the extension of Western education. The Italians believed that provision of Western-type education was one of the most effective ways of winning over the subject people. However, the main objective of the Italian educational effort was geared towards Italianisation, not academic advancement. Amharic was the only language taught in schools; this policy marginalised the teaching of Ge'ez, which was of central importance to church-based medical education.[49] After the restoration of Ethiopia's independence, many church-educated individuals were employed in Western-style schools to teach Amharic, while the emperor for his part continued to encourage church scholars to translate Ge'ez religious texts into Amharic, further reducing the need for students to learn Ge'ez.[50] Interest in Ge'ez continued to decline in the post-Italian period; partly because the church failed to ensure that language was included in the new national curriculum. Thus the new generation of Ethiopian students learning in European-type schools had no access to Ge'ez. The inability of students to gain access to it, in which much church-based medical knowledge was preserved, threatened the sustainability of that knowledge.

Conclusion

The restoration of the country's independence in May 1941 boosted the morale of church-educated healers and encouraged them to resume their duties to deliver multi-faceted medico-magical services to a cross-section of the Ethiopian public in a spirit of freedom. Following the end of the Italian occupation, the Ministry of Interior, recognising the potential for indigenous medicine to enhance the welfare of the country's population, issued a proclamation in 1942,[51] permitting indigenous healers to work as healthcare providers. This measure was reinforced by the Ministry of Public Health's proclamation of the late 1940s in which indigenous health practitioners were required to register and have a work permit.[52] The imperial government's support of indigenous medicine was, in part, a gesture towards preserving the country's cultural heritage, and partly an expression of its support for the anti-colonialist nationalist sentiment that was beginning to spread across the African continent. These legal provisions guaranteed a limited working space to indigenous healers, including cleric–healers; but the administration of the registration system, along with the attitudes of Western medical authorities, limited the degree to which indigenous healing practitioners were able to operate freely within the changing medical marketplace of the 1950s and 1960s. By contrast, the limitations of the Western-based healthcare system provided opportunities for other types of healers, including the 'injectionists', to work as competitors of allopathic health practitioners, and church-based healers, ensuring that therapeutic pluralism continued to be a feature of the post-Italian medical landscape.

The medical marketplace in the post-Italian period saw limited expansion of biomedical institutions. Yet this expansion failed to keep up with the exponential growth in demand for health services by the great majority of the population. The access to healthcare facilities, moreover, became entangled in a web of bureaucratic and administrative problems, making them incapable of offering organised preventative or curative services or of dislodging the entrenched position of indigenous medicine. Examining the position of healers during the post-Italian era in view of the state's efforts to legalise indigenous medicine and the state structures that limited the ability of indigenous healers to function freely is of vital importance. The book will look into this important subject in the following chapters.

Figure 10: Protective amulet against spirit of darkness

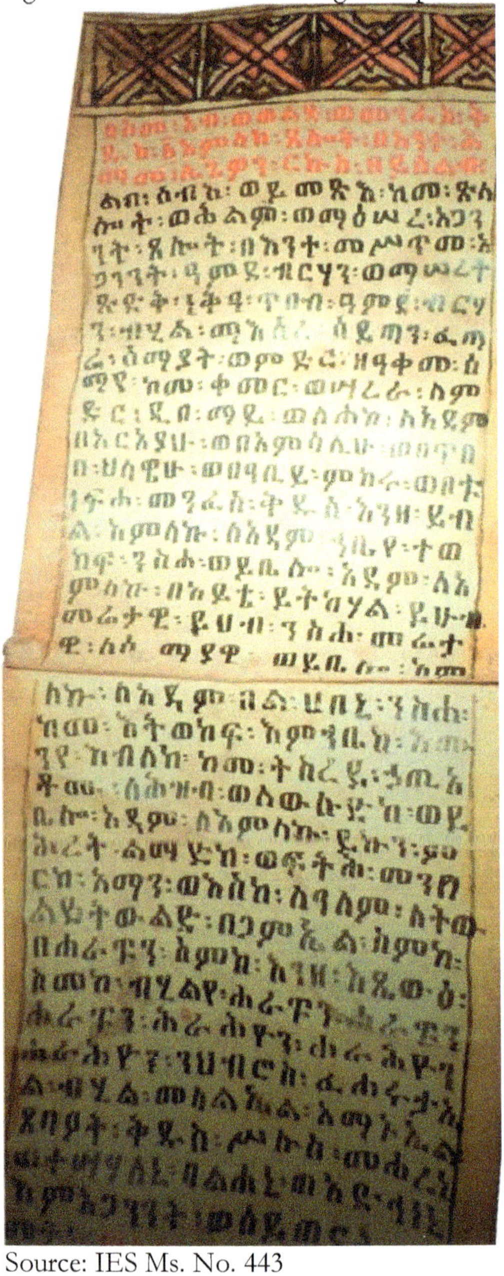

Source: IES Ms. No. 443

Figure 11: Talismanic drawing to fend off or frighten malicious spirits

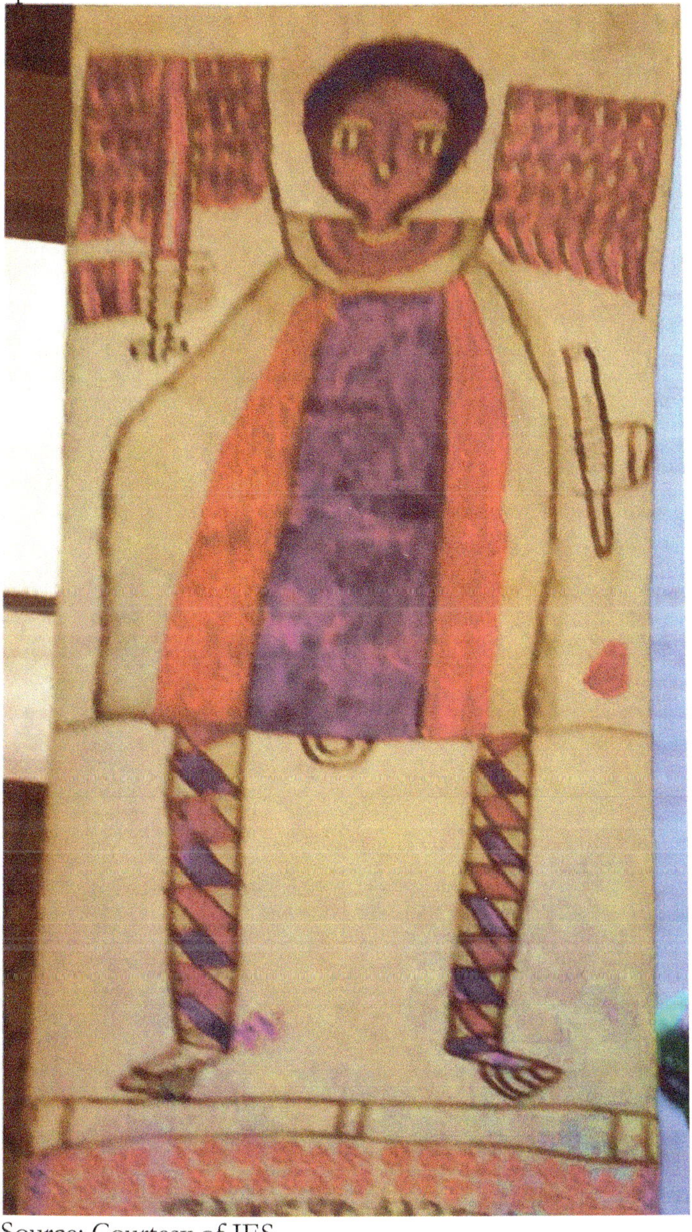

Source: Courtesy of IES

Figure 12: A magical amulet for personal use

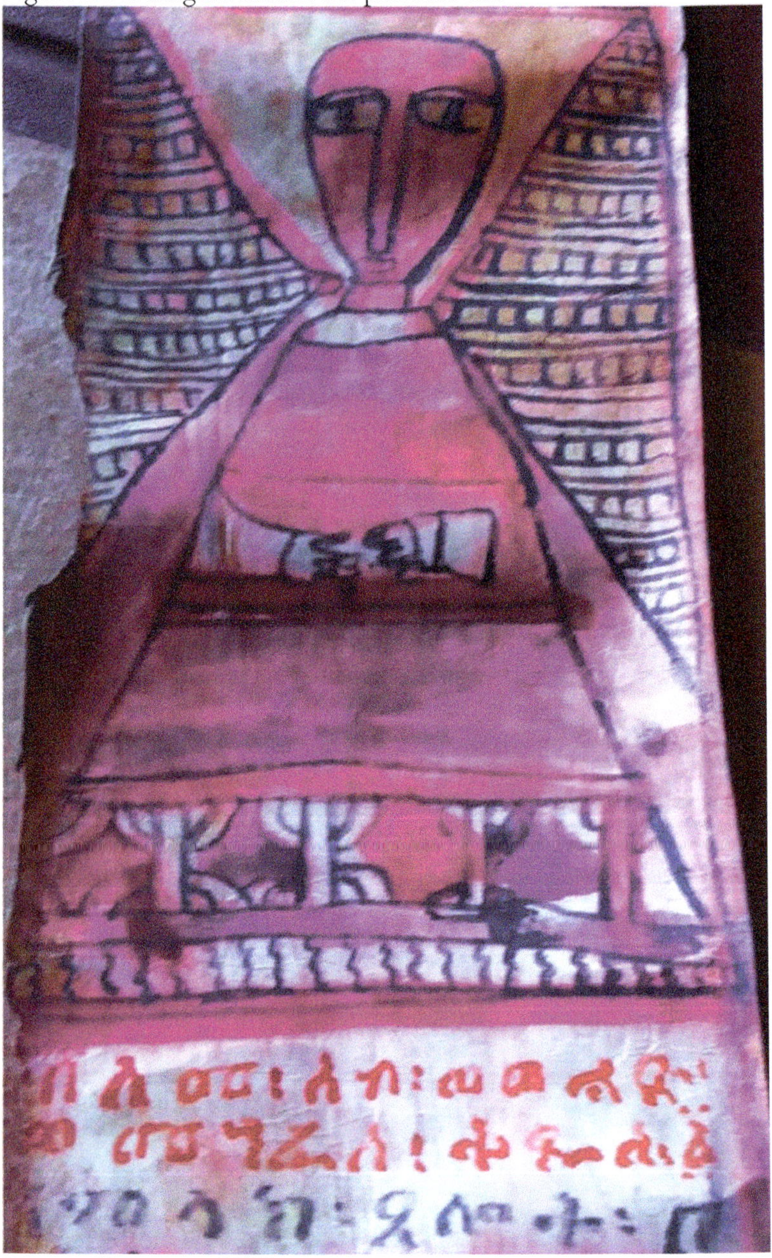

Source: Courtesy of IES

Notes

1 Richard Pankhurst, 'Some Notes for the History of Typhus,' *Mimeograph*, 1975, 11.

2 Ibid., 12.

3 This measure may also have been introduced to prevent miscegenation, discourage the Italian army from drifting towards same-sex relationships and to maintain its fighting spirit.

4 Assefa Nega, 'Malaria', in *The Ecology of Health and Disease in Ethiopia*, edited by Helmut Kloos and Zein Ahmed Zein (Colorado: Westview Press, 1993), 341.

5 Frank Shorter, *The Conquest of Malaria, Italy, 1900–1962* (New Haven: Yale University Press, 2006); Randall Packard, *The Making of a Tropical Disease: A Short History of Malaria* (Baltimore: The Johns Hopkins University Press, 2007), 128–131.

6 Andrew J. Carlson and Dennis G. Carlson, *Health, Wealth, and Family in Rural Ethiopia: Kossoye, North Gondar Region, 1963–2007*, (Addis Ababa: Addis Ababa University Press, 2008), 91.

7 Richard Pankhurst, 'The Medical History of Ethiopia During the Italian Invasion and Occupation (1935–1941)' *Journal of Ethiopian Studies*, 4(2): (1973): 111.

8 As noted by Dr Asrat, the first post-liberation surgeon, the popularity of *calcio* may have increased the acceptability of biomedical treatments with hypodermic needles. See Asrat Waldayes, 'The Postliberation Period (1941–1973)', in *An Introduction to the Medical History of Ethiopia*, edited by Richard Pankhurst (Trenton: The Red Sea Press, 1990), 245.

9 Ibid.

10 Habte Mariam Workineh, 'Teaching of the Ethiopian Orthodox Church on Matters Related to Health and Disease', *An Introduction to Health and Heath Education in Ethiopia*, compiled and edited by E. Fuller Torrey (Addis Ababa: Artistic Printers, 1967), 89.

11 F.O. 371, No. 41498, A Report by A. F. Mathew, October 1943.

12 Spencer Trimingham, *Islam in Ethiopia* (London: Clarendon Press, 1952), 137.

13 Yet, the extent to which this pro-Muslim Italian policy was applied differed from place to place; unlike the predominantly Muslim-inhabited areas, the colonial officials, for instance, were not truly committed to promoting Muslims to higher positions of power in the overwhelmingly Christian-dominated regions. For a comprehensive discussion of Italian colonial policy in Ethiopia, see Alberto Sbacchi, *Ethiopia Under Mussolini: Fascism and the Colonial Experience* (London: Zed Books, 1985).

14 Ibid.

15 He was one of the first five Ethiopian Archbishops anointed by the Alexandrian Patriarch in 1929. Mersha Alelegn, *A Brief Biography of Ethiopian Bishops* (Amharic) (Addis Ababa: Ethio Tikur Abbay Printers, 2005), 74.

16 Haile Selassie, *My Life and Ethiopia's Progress*, vol. 2 (Amharic), (Addis Ababa: Berhanena Selam Printing Press, 1966, E.C.), 53–54.

17 Alberto Sbacchi, *Legacy of Bitterness: Ethiopia and Fascist Italy, 1935-1941* (New Jersey: The Red Sea Press, 1997), 171.

18 For a partial list of religious institutions that had been ransacked or destroyed by the Italians in Shewa, see the voluminous text on the biography of religious figures, and the history of churches and monasteries edited by Daniel Kibret (Ed.), *Church Documents*, vol. 1 (Amharic) (Addis Ababa: Mega Printing Enterprise, 1999, E.C.).

19 John Markakis, *Ethiopia: Anatomy of a Traditional Polity* (Oxford: Oxford University Press, 1974), 146.

20 See Alberto Sbacchi, *Ethiopia Under Mussolini*, 194.

21 Oral informants have also espoused a different view about the Italian attack on church-based healers. They argued that the Italians were 'knowledgeable occultists and they had every reason to target church-based healers, the ones who could figure out and expose the true intentions of the colonial authorities'. Since the Italians targeted quite a few church-educated elites, it is not surprising to find such ordeals inflicted upon cleric–healers during the occupation period.

22 Richard Pankhurst, 'Italian Fascist War Crimes in Ethiopia: History of Their Discussion, from the League of Nations to the United Nations (1936–1949)," *Northeast African Studies*, 6(1–2) (1999): 83.

23 Ministry of Interior, file no. 29/63, Abebe Desta to the Ministry of Interior, n.d July 1942.

24 Alberto Sbacchi, *Ethiopia Under Mussolini*, 194.

25 Oral informants nos. 23, 34, 35, 39 and 43.

26 Fantahun Engeda, *Major Political Problems and Struggles during Haile Selassie's Administration as Learned from the Biography of the Emperor's Close Associates* (Amharic) (Addis Ababa: Berhanena Selam Printing Press, 1997, E.C.), 106.

27 Bahru Zewde, *A History of Modern Ethiopia 1855–1974* (Addis Ababa: Addis Ababa University Press, 1991), 172.

28 Alberto Sbacchi, *Ethiopia Under Mussolini*, 194.

29 In the words of Sbacchi, 'Before it was proved that the actors of the plot had sought refuge at the monastery [of Dabre Libanos], Graziani intended to disband the institute of religious studies and prevent the gathering of students.' Ibid., 195.

30 Ian Campbell, *The Plot to Kill Graziani: The Attempted Assassination of Mussolini's Viceroy* (Addis Ababa: Addis Ababa University Press, 2010), p.319.
31 Paul Henze, 'Movement toward Modernization: A Century of Progress', in *Layers of Time: A History of Ethiopia*, edited by Helmut Kloos and Zein Ahmed Zein (London, Hurst & Co., 2000), 327.
32 Spencer Trimingham, *Islam in Ethiopia*, 137.
33 Paul Henze, 'Movement Toward Modernization', 11.
34 Anonymous, *The Patriots' Struggle against the Fascists* (Amharic), (Addis Ababa: Berhanena Selam Printing Press, 1941, E.C.), 23.
35 Paul Henze, 'Movement Toward Modernization', 11.
36 Ibid. See also Ministry of Interior, file no. 4/2, G. G. Campbell, Director-General of Medical Services, 'Memorandum for the U.N.R.R.A. Mission to Ethiopia', 11 February 1946.
37 Bahru Zewde, *A History of Modern Ethiopia*, 164.
38 Richard Pankhurst, 'The Medical History of Ethiopia During the Italian Invasion and Occupation (1935–1941)', 113–114.
39 Treatment of the sick with anti-bacterial drugs was the only known therapy in the post-Italian period. It may be argued that the recent introduction of the last two venereal diseases was the likely reason why church-based healers could not figure out the nature of these diseases or incorporate some therapeutically valuable items in local medical texts. However, in the case of *bambulie*, secular healers known as the *waggesha* or 'surgeon–herbalists' were the ones who came to the aid of afflicted individuals; other than easing the pain by removing abscess and cauterising the swollen genital area, the *waggesha* did not provide any known herbal or other medication therapies.
40 Mesele Terecha kebede, *Leprosy, Leprosaria and Society in Ethiopia* (Addis Ababa: The Armaeur Hansen Research Institute, 2008), 63.
41 Many local oral stories about the Italian crimes committed against lepers exist.
42 Sebastian O'Kelly, *Amedeo: The True Story of An Italian's War in Abyssinia* (London: Harper Collins Publishers, 2003), 101.
43 Harold Marcus, *A History of Ethiopia* (Berkeley: University of California Press, 1994), 150.
44 F.O. 371, no. 41498, A Report by A. F. Mathew, October 1943.
45 Alberto Sbacchi, *Ethiopia Under Mussolini*, 194.
46 For a contemporaneous account by a non-Amhara writer of this Italian effort, see Hiywot Hedaru, *Those Days Have Been Forgotten: From School to Consular Work 1932–1941* (Amharic) (Addis Ababa: Berhanena Selam Printing Press, 1967, E.C.), 12. See also Tilahun Berhane Selassie,

Twentieth Century Ethiopia, vol. 1 (Amharic) (Addis Ababa: Artistic Printing Press, 1998, E.C.), 400.

47 Its Amharic rendering reads: [ሕዝቡ] ... ሌላ የዓለማዊ[ና] ፖለቲካ ትምህርት የሌላቸው ስለሆኑ መነኮሳት ወይም ባሕታዊያን በዚህ ዘመን እንደዚህ ይሆናል ብለው ሲነግሯቸው ከእግዚአብሄር የተላኩ እየመሰላቸው እውነት አድርገው ይቀበላሉና በዚህም ለመጠቀም ኢጣልያኖች ይህን ስለ ዐወቁ ዋና መሣርያ አድርገውት ነበር።። Haile Selassie, *My Life and Ethiopia's Progress*, vol. 1 (Amharic) (Addis Ababa: Berhanena Selam Printing Press, 1965, E.C.), 134.

48 Alberto Sbacchi, *Legacy of Bitterness*, 179.

49 Chris Prouty and Eugene Rosenfeld, *Historical Dictionary of Ethiopia* (Metuchen & London: The Scarecrow Press, 1981), 55.

50 In 1918, after summoning a group of church scholars, the regent ordered them to translate and prepare religious texts in both Ge'ez and Amharic, the result of which was to be published as of 1922 by Berhanena Selam, a state-owned printing press. See Sergew Hable Selassie (Ed.), 'Amharic Church Dictionary', Institute of Ethiopian Studies, unpublished manuscript (n.d). For a list of church scholars and scribes involved in the translation and copying of religious texts, see Berihun Kebede, *History of Emperor Haile Selassie* (Amharic) (Addis Ababa: Artistic Printing Press, 1993, E.C.), 317–323.

51 See, Article 8 of Proclamation no. 27 of 1942.

52 Ministry of Health, file no. ቀ-9, n.d. See also Proclamation no. 100 of September 1948, Imperial Ethiopian Government, *Negarit Gazeta*, sub-article 3 (B), 1948.

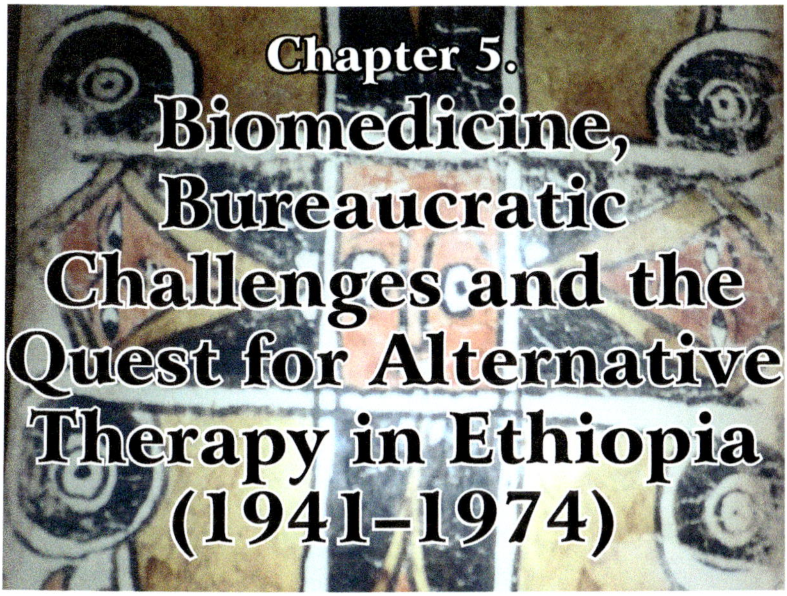

Chapter 5. Biomedicine, Bureaucratic Challenges and the Quest for Alternative Therapy in Ethiopia (1941–1974)

The end of the Italian occupation and the restoration of the Ethiopian monarchy transformed the medical marketplace in Ethiopia, shifting the balance between practitioners of Western biomedicine and various forms of indigenous healing. The Italians had increased the number of hospitals and medical practitioners in Ethiopia, and launched a number of public health campaigns. They had also attacked various indigenous healing professions as part of their efforts to squash resistance to their occupation. These moves had weakened the hold that indigenous healers had had on the Ethiopian population. With the end of the occupation, however, many of the Western medical practitioners left the country and hospitals fell into disrepair. The British forces, who played a critical role in dislodging the Italians in 1941, had little interest in investing in the development of a more effective health system. At the same time, the social disruption created by the efforts to dislodge the Italians from the country contributed to a rise in the prevalence of disease in many parts of the country.

Declining health services and rising disease burdens created space for indigenous health practitioners, including cleric–healers, to reassert their role as principal healthcare providers. They were encouraged in this effort by the Imperial Ethiopian Government, which had regained full control of the country in 1944 and, at least on paper, had adopted the view that indigenous practitioners needed to play an important role in meeting the health needs of the Ethiopian people.

This chapter explores the health policies of the restored imperial government and the manifold bureaucratic/administrative problems that beleaguered their efforts to expand the biomedical healthcare system from the end of the Italian interlude to the 1974 revolution. It also investigates how the limits of Western healthcare coverage provided space within which various forms of indigenous healing could function and for the emergence of new forms of hybrid medical care, including that provided by a growing number of so-called injectionists. Consequently, the Ethiopian people seeking medical treatment during the imperial era picked up their therapeutic preference(s) from within a highly pluralistic health system, similar to those described by Janzen in Lower Zaire and Good in Kenya.[1]

The Limits of Western Medical Care

The British military administration that was set up after the defeat of the Italians in 1941 temporarily replaced the Italian rule in Ethiopia. With the conclusion of the 1942 and 1944 Anglo-Ethiopian agreements, Ethiopia's national sovereignty was re-established. Freed from British control, Emperor Haile Selassie embarked on advancing 'the goals he had set when he first came to power in the 1920s: consolidation of the central government, expansion of infrastructure for economic development, spread of educational opportunities, and creation of strong professional military and police forces.'[2] Haile Selassie's government was also committed to improvements in health as part of this larger development scheme. While the government achieved some success in fulfilling many of these goals, improving the health system proved difficult to achieve. As a result, the government was unable to reduce the country's disease burden, which had been increasing since the end of the Italian occupation.[3]

The inability of the public health system to improve the health of the population encouraged the public to continue seeking therapeutic services from church-based and other indigenous healers.

The huge cost of reconstruction, including the provision of new healthcare infrastructure, was a formidable challenge to the restored government.[4] The Ministry of Interior, which was entrusted to look after health matters, possessed limited human and material resources. Moreover, the ministry operated through a bureaucratic system that was plagued by red tape which stymied it from responding to the country's health problems in a timely and efficient manner.[5]

Shortages in medical facilities and staff were a very serious problem facing the government. It began establishing health centres in the 1950s and the number of government clinics grew from 28 in 1934 to 105 in 1954. During the same period, the number of hospitals grew to 38. Yet this growth still left the population underserved. The government's goal of having a district health centre per 50 000 people was not achieved until the 1970s. Moreover, there were only 80 physicians in the country in 1954. Nearly all of them were foreigners, including a substantial number of missionary doctors. There were only a few Ethiopian physicians, all of whom were graduates of foreign universities. To staff the health centres, the first public health college was founded in Gondar in 1954. Additional training institutions for nurses, health assistants, health officers, sanitarians and pharmacists were established in the 1970s. The first medical school was established in Addis Ababa in the early 1960s.

The country also lacked an adequate system for disease reporting. Provincial governors were primarily responsible for assessing and reporting disease outbreaks to the Minister of Interior, coordinating the available medical services at their disposals, and taking any decisive measure deemed necessary to fight against the scourges that affected the people of their provinces, including requesting assistance from the central government. The governors, in turn, only received information on disease outbreaks once it had been funnelled up through a complex administrative hierarchy of local authorities.

The *cheqa shum* (village headmen) were often the first to report the outbreak of a disease. They could not, however, communicate this information directly to the provincial governor. Instead, they were required to communicate the news to the deputy district (*woreda*) governors (*mikitil woreda ghezie* or *meslane*)[6] who then reported the outbreak to district governors (*woreda ghezie*). The *woreda* governors passed the information to the sub-provincial or *awraja* governors (*awraja ghezie*), who communicated with the provincial governors (*teklay ghezie*; also known as *endarassie*, literally meaning 'on my behalf').[7] Not surprisingly, the need to pass information through this complex hierarchy of local officials created a serious barrier to the timely reporting of disease outbreaks to the Minister of Interior's office.[8] A report of a *cheqa shum* might take weeks to pass through *woreda* and *awraja* officials in order to reach the provincial governor's office. Once there, moreover, a similar delay could also occur before the provincial governor passed the information on to the health unit in the Ministry of Interior, an office entrusted to review the report and act accordingly.[9]

Further delays could occur after notification of the outbreak of a disease had reached the Ministry of Interior. The minister's office was inundated with requests for immediate medical supplies and personnel. The minister could not, even if he wanted to, respond to all these requests in a timely manner. As a result, the ministry's first response to requests for aid was often to remind the provincial and district governors that such requests should reach its office only when the existing healthcare facilities in their districts could not cope with reported health problems.[10] The ministry also reprimanded administrative officials for not mobilising the available resources at their disposal before they requested additional medical assistance.

The Minister of Interior was also handicapped in his efforts to respond appropriately to requests for medical aid, by the poor-quality and sometimes exaggerated nature of the reports he received. Lack of access to biomedically trained health personnel frequently led administrative officials to submit inaccurate reports to their superiors. To deal with this ubiquitous problem, the Wallo clinic administration proposed that the provincial governor's office assess the feasibility of deploying persons of some biomedical knowledge to the *woreda* level and supporting them through the allocation of agricultural lands in lieu of their salary.[11]

Most of the time, the languages used in the reports to describe signs and symptoms of diseases did not provide a clear picture of what kind of health problem the local officials faced. The manner of describing the illnesses was no better than the languages customarily used by ordinary people or, at best, that of indigenous healers.

Absence of 'differential diagnosis of acute febrile illnesses'[12] was among the many problems in disease reporting; for instance, relapsing fever was often misdiagnosed as louse-borne typhus. This led to calls for typhus vaccinations which, when administered, failed to provide protection.[13]

Occasionally, misreporting of epidemics served other purposes; for example, local administrators in Wore Himano district in Wallo made an urgent appeal for medical supplies and personnel to deal with an unidentified communicable disease outbreak in 1966. It was subsequently discovered that this outbreak had been fuelled by a prolonged drought and famine that had not been reported. Reporting the outbreak as a distinct and unrelated misfortune appeared to have been a deliberate attempt by local administrative officials to hide the famine situation. An exchange of accusations followed between the provincial governorate, which blamed the severity of the outbreak on the failure of the Ministry of Health to respond quickly to requests for assistance, and the Ministry of Health which laid responsibility on the governorate for not dealing with the drought and famine. After much correspondence and a lapse of considerable time, the Ministry of Interior finally suggested that 'distribution of relief food alongside medicine' was the only solution to ease the fear and despair of the famished population.[14] In most cases information coming from 'lower-level administrators' was often 'too fragmentary, general, unintelligible and unconvincing to those above', whose 'questions [for clarification for confirmation] and instructions were also incomprehensible and impractical to the lower officials.'[15]

The ministry repeatedly demanded that administrative officials accurately report the diseases that they felt required immediate medical intervention. This meant identifying the affected areas, the overall nature and outward manifestations of the diseases, along with the kind of medical assistance they wished to obtain. In addition, they were told that before conveying their reports to the ministry, provincial and district officials should send health practitioners to the affected localities to verify the reports that came from lower-level officials. Responsible officials or their delegates were also required to assist health workers in dealing with the reported health problems.[16]

In an effort to reduce the flood of inaccurate reports of disease outbreaks further, the Ministry of Interior, which at times requested bizarre details (e.g., 'names of the people who had died of famine' or 'a sample of the rats' that had destroyed crops),[17] adopted a policy of penalising local administrators for unsubstantiated reports. The ministry wrote: '[E]very local governor should be aware of reimbursing all the expenses incurred if the reported cases proved untrue.'[18]

Local authorities tried their best to meet the ministry's reporting requirements. One means of doing this was to utilise the mobile health teams that the ministry sent to the provinces to investigate potential outbreaks. The ministry supported this use of health personnel as long as the teams provided daily reports of their activities and the local authority agreed to cover their expenses.[19] The Wallo provincial governorate office, at the insistence of a certain Dr J. Pavars, an administrator of the government hospital in Dessie, requested that the Ministry of Health assign a mobile public health team or anti-epidemic unit[20] to the whole province on a permanent basis.[21] If the request was not rejected, the wished-for units in the provinces could have initiated the founding of 'epidemic-prevention centres' equipped to conduct immunisation works and to educate the rural people in disease-prevention methods.

While the ministry supported health investigations, it sought to limit the abuse of this service by insisting that local authorities cover the expenses of such inquiries if they found no cases. Thus, the ministry warned a provincial hospital administrator, who had requested health workers to investigate outbreaks in remote localities, only to be told by the investigators that no patients were to be found,[22] that in future requests for health investigations would only be considered, 'if and only if district governorate offices are willing to cover all the daily expenses of the health personnel and transportation costs'.[23]

While mobile health units could help local authorities investigate disease outbreaks, the effectiveness of the teams was limited by the absence of transportation facilities in rural areas and other problems, including attacks from local bandits.[24] Incidents of robbery and physical attacks were very common and lower-level authorities were constantly reminded about the need to provide armed escorts to mobile health teams sent to their *woreda*s or localities. Many rural localities, lacking even bumpy dry-weather roads, could not be accessed with the sturdiest of vehicles. The problem only increased during the rainy seasons when the foot trails became muddy and rivers overflowed their banks.

The need to identify the cause of disease outbreaks accurately led one local administrator to propose that sick cases be transported by motor vehicle to the nearest health facility for diagnosis. Though this was a potentially valuable suggestion, the Ministry of Interior rejected it, arguing that deadly diseases could be rapidly transmitted to disease-free areas. It is also obvious that the suggestion was impractical due to the poor condition of the roads in many rural areas.

For their part, the members of mobile health units sometimes felt that their services had been misused when they struggled to reach remote localities only to find a few non-contagious cases or no patients at all. Health workers also expressed their disappointment when they discovered that the epidemic they had been sent to investigate turned out to be a case where the domestic servant of a local governor had fallen ill.[25]

The use of medical personnel to investigate the outbreaks of disease posed another problem. It drew health workers away from clinical work and, as a result, many patients were unable to get medical assistance from government clinics or they had to wait for days to receive treatment.[26]

The provision of Western biomedical health services during the imperial era was also hampered by jurisdictional conflicts between the provincial government offices and the health unit of the Ministry of Interior, which became a separate Ministry of Public Health in 1948. The new ministry saw itself as having primary responsibility for health matters. However, chief provincial governors, and through them the Minister of Interior, retained the 'power of supervision over all governmental agencies at the provincial level and the authority to give orders to officials of all branches of government at that level'; which included the authority to supervise health activities.[27] Thus when requesting medical assistance from the Ministry of Public Health, provincial administrative officials were required to send copies of their requisitions to the Ministry of Interior as well. Moreover, all requests needed to observe the bureaucratic chain of command, which meant requests for medical assistance had to be communicated through the provincial health departments and clinic administrations, along with the endorsement of local administrative offices, all of which fell under the Ministry of Interior.[28] Local officials, who tried to request help directly from the Ministry of Public Health, were rebuffed and told that all requests needed to come through the official bureaucratic hierarchy. Thus, despite the creation of a separate Ministry of Public Health, the various provincial administrative offices continued to exercise their control over health-related matters in the 1960s. This pattern did not significantly change even when Ethiopian health professionals and physicians, numbering about 23 in 1964,[29] began to administer hospitals and provincial health offices for the first time.[30]

Overall, the combination of the lack of health centres, trained personnel and good communications networks, including the absence of all-weather roads, and the necessity of working through a complex bureaucratic hierarchy (in an over-bureaucratised and over-centralised system) in which multiple officials exercised authority, prevented the effective and timely provision of Western medical care over wide areas of Ethiopia.

According to health workers, the provision of Western biomedicine in Ethiopia was also hampered by local attitudes towards health care. They reported having difficulty propagating biomedical ideas because 'unscientific' medical beliefs were deeply rooted among the public; for example, a health assistant in Wallo noted that local populations believed that typhus was conveyed directly from one person to another. As a consequence, they feared caring for typhus patients, believing that they would catch the disease just by talking to, or looking at, the patients.[31] Many patients died of lack of food and water. In addition, local populations did not report the disease to local health officials, preventing them from responding to the needs of typhus-afflicted areas.

Even when medical assistance was made available, people were not always ready to take advantage of it. Most of the time, the ingestion of pills was not a preferred mode of treatment, partly because it was equated with taking unknown food that contradicted their religious beliefs. By contrast, the enthusiasm for the injection needle, which had been widely used during the Italian occupation, continued. According to the Ministry of Health, injections were received as a valid and wonder-working mode of treatment in almost all cases of transmissible and epidemic diseases, such as typhus, typhoid and relapsing fever, pneumonia, bacillus or amoebic dysentery.[32]

However, people were less passionate about prophylactic vaccines given to them with a hypodermic needle. The director in the Ministry of Health wrote in the 1950s that vaccinations against smallpox and typhus were administered freely but people were unenthusiastic about being vaccinated.[33] Often, providing vaccines without the assistance of administrative organs was almost impossible. Despite the issuance of scores of government regulations and notices, the degree of acceptance of prophylaxes in the mid-twentieth century was low. In the case of smallpox, for example, the rural masses, for the most part, continued to rely on variolation, which had been practised in Ethiopia since at least the eighteenth century. This involved the use of pus from a smallpox patient to immunise a healthy individual.[34] Some people also refused to allow their infected children to receive medical treatment, believing that the disease-causing spirit would be offended if the sick were given any injectable treatment. This indigenous outlook lingered until the eradication of smallpox in Ethiopia in the late 1970s.

The health system was also handicapped by marked inequalities in the distribution of health facilities. While urban areas were relatively well served, rural areas continued to have few facilities. This imbalance led a number of governors to call for the building of new health facilities in their districts; for example, while corresponding with higher authorities the provincial governor of Wallo, an exceptionally enlightened *endarassie* (literally 'on behalf of me') frequently noted the scarcity of public health institutions in his province. One of the arguments he employed to support his request for more facilities was the discrepancy between the amount of health taxes he collected[35] and the health budget earmarked for his province. According to his calculation, about 650 914.71 birr in health taxes was collected from his province every year, while only 327 629 birr was allocated as a health budget and the remaining 323 290.71 birr was poured into the coffers of the central government.

The governor underscored the fact that the handing over of almost 50% of the health tax to the central government created a huge budget deficit that put his administration in a precarious financial position and halted him from providing medical care to the tax-paying people of the province. The *endarassie*, explaining the depressing situation that prevailed in his province, wrote: 'The majority of people are living in complete darkness and in remote localities that required them to travel up to fifteen days to get to the clinics; they cannot even afford to buy Aspirin and are totally helpless without the services of traditional medical practitioners.'[36]

Part of the tax problem lay in the fact that despite legal provisions which stated that '[t]he health taxes collected by the Ministry of Finance and appropriated to the Ministry of Public Health shall be expended by the said ministry for the purpose of expanding and improving public health facilities throughout the Empire',[37] the ministry had no authority to enforce these provisions, as responsibility for doing something about the health taxes was in the hands of an Advisory Board of Health constituting the Minister of Health and five other high-ranking individuals hand-picked by the Emperor.[38] Thus in the end, the provision of health services depended on lengthy consultations between the Ministry of Health and the Imperial Court. Unfortunately, the emperor who appeared more interested in boosting his paternal benevolent image than in meeting the health needs of his subjects, preferred to establish biomedical institutions that would be administered under a charitable organisation named after him.[39] The recurring appeals of provincial governors for healthcare facilities most often went unanswered.

Had provincial advisory councils been entrusted with real executive power, provincial governors, including the energetic *endarassie* of Wallo, could have established more than a few public health facilities in their dominions. It is worth indicating that the dearth of biomedical establishments, an intractable problem attributable partly to the Ministry of Health's lack of authority to administer health taxes, was not the only obstacle that prevented common people from accessing preventive and curative medical services.

Another pivotal issue was the imperial government's policy regarding the development of the private health sector in Ethiopia. During the 1940s and 1950s, allopathic health practitioners, who were almost entirely foreign nationals, were permitted to engage in private medical practice. However, in the 1960s, at the time when Ethiopian doctors had begun to join the medical profession, the Ministry of Health made it hard for biomedical practitioners to take on part-time private medical activities.[40] A circular letter that came into effect in August 1964 banned biomedical practitioners from working in private clinics.[41] This prohibition was aimed particularly at encouraging Ethiopians, whose education had been funded by the state, to work within the public health sector.[42] The circular claimed that

> many medical practitioners have taken advantage of [the lack of qualified medical practitioners in the country] . . . and have tried to fill this vacuum by dispensing private medical services in private clinics and private places . . . the government is entitled to [look over] the full-time services of medical practitioners it employs and is bound to prevent acts which are prejudicial to the rights and interests of patients for whose benefit the medical practitioners are employed.[43]

The policy was intended to prevent the drain of trained medical personnel from the public sector. However, in the absence of adequate public health institutions, the ban on biomedical practitioners working in private practice had the overall effect of limiting the expansion of Western-oriented medical care in the country.

The provision of Western biomedical care by the Ethiopian government was supplemented by the building of medical mission hospitals. However, the government claimed that mission hospitals refused to work with public healthcare facilities during outbreaks of epidemics. Referring to one of the articles signed between the Ministry of Health and foreign medical missions, the ministry reminded the latter that they had to comply with the agreement and make contributions of health workers (not medicines) whenever and wherever epidemic diseases broke out.[44] For Talbot, a one-time editor-in-chief of the government daily, *Ethiopian Herald*, repeated appeals for medical assistance strained relations between government and mission-run medical facilities.[45]

As shown above, the existing biomedical facilities proved inadequate to the needs of the increasing population. This situation did little to encourage people to seek out biomedical care. Local health authorities, for their part, saw this reluctance as resulting from the presence of indigenous healers, and particularly injectionists, whom they viewed as competing for their patients. Almost all government-owned clinics favoured regulations prohibiting not only those who administered injections, but also the few drug shops that retailed 'inappropriate and even expired medicaments'.[46]

In a situation where Western health services were not adequately distributed and peoples' perception about their efficacy, while varying significantly from illness to illness, was generally low, it is not surprising that the population often turned to alternative therapeutic resources, including church-based healers.

Western medical practitioners, for their part, saw church healers as serving important medical functions which complemented the use of biomedical healing resources; for example, indigenous 'psychotherapy' was seen as particularly vital for dealing with most psycho-social illnesses,[47] In addition, many idiopathic illnesses, the bane of Western practitioners, were routinely referred to cleric/spiritual healers. Indigenous healers were also viewed as effective in 'influencing the emotional and spiritual aspects of health probably through the power of suggestion'.[48] Biomedical practitioners recognised that they were ill-equipped to appreciate the indigenous medical beliefs and the psycho-social perspective of illness causations.

Yet people's decision to employ non-Western medical resources did not fit easily into the complementary categories imagined by Western trained physicians. Instead, they sought out alternative therapies for a wide range of health problems, including many illnesses Western medical authorities claimed to be able to treat. In some cases, people resisted consulting physicians because Western illness labels, diagnoses and treatments were incompatible or even contradictory, with indigenous beliefs. They also claimed that practitioners of Western allopathic medicine could not effectively communicate with them or understand the underlying causes of their problems.[49] This created communication barriers between biomedical practitioners and their patients.[50]

The Quest for Alternative Therapy

The limitations of Western medicine following the end of the Italian occupation created space for a range of alternative therapies to thrive. These included church-based healers and other forms of indigenous therapy that had a long history in Ethiopia. No longer persecuted, and officially acknowledged by the state, various forms of healing thrived during the imperial era. It would be a mistake, however, to view these alternative therapies as simply vestiges of earlier forms of therapy. New forms of therapy that combined indigenous medical knowledge with allopathic medical practices, particularly the use of injections, emerged during this period. In addition, older forms of indigenous therapeutics underwent transformations in response to changing social conditions, including the growth of literacy and the proliferation of printing technology. In the remainder of this chapter, an endeavour has been made to examine the history of injectionists and other practitioners who combined Western biomedical treatments with indigenous ideas and practices.

The Role of the Injectionists

The failure of the public health system to tackle both endemic and epidemic diseases in the post Italian period, combined with the growing popularity of injections, created an opportunity in Ethiopia, as elsewhere in Africa, for individuals who administered injections to position themselves as biomedically trained practitioners. By emphasising the alleged efficacy of their healing strategies, which were based on a mix of Western and indigenous ideas about disease causation, the injectionists had little difficulty attracting clients. Injectionists have become a pervasive part of the African medical landscape, yet little research has been done on their history.

The rural public sought the services of the injectionists, in part, because they filled a gap in the biomedical system. For most rural households, the decision to visit a healthcare facility was a difficult one; distance, medical and transport costs, not to mention time and personal expenses, were serious challenges that discouraged the majority of the rural masses from tapping the existing biomedical facilities. In most instances a family with few household resources could not afford to pay for such a costly trip. Even those who could afford to pay for treatments often had to do so by sacrificing other essential household spending, which would naturally result in the depletion of the assets of already impoverished households. No less serious, many people resisted making large financial sacrifices to attend a healthcare institution that they viewed as providing inadequate care. For all these people, injectionists were often close at hand and provided a medical service that most people viewed as efficacious. In addition, the injectionists shared common etiological concepts with their patients, and blended their use of injections and antibiotics with local healing practices.[51]

While injectionists were popular among the people, cleric–healers scorned those who blended indigenous and biomedical products. Cleric healers viewed these 'hybrid' healers as indecent practitioners whose principal motive was to exploit the credulity of the common people to their own advantage. Cleric–healers held 'hybrid' healers accountable for dishonouring genuine practitioners, offering their services without a taint of hypocrisy; these ill-motivated and insincere practitioners conspicuously assisted those who wanted to defame and discredit indigenous therapeutics. The unfounded claims of 'hybrid' healers as skilled practitioners of indigenous and Western medicine also contributed to the view of health officials that all alternative healthcare providers were quacks or unqualified.[52]

Cleric–healers claimed that the injectionists' use of resources from both indigenous and biomedicine reflected their lack of knowledge of either therapeutic system. Needless to say, cleric–healers also viewed injectionists as threatening their financial interests by drawing away patients. As a result, the majority of cleric–healers called for the prohibition and eviction of 'hybrid' healers from the medical marketplace.

Trained biomedical practitioners criticised the problem of healers using and abusing antibiotics and injections from the immediate post-Italian period through to the early 1970s. 'Injectionists', whom biomedical health personnel sarcastically called 'itinerant village doctors', were accused of unlawful medical practices and distracting the people from using allopathic medicine.[53] However, the government health workers were also concerned about loss of revenue. The head of a newly established government clinic (a clinic operating only for a little more than two months)[54] wrote that the injectionists and an illegal rural drug shop were drawing patients away from his clinic, making it impossible for the clinic to provide biomedical services to the local community. His report, which may have exaggerated the actual state of affairs in order to gain the attention of higher authorities, stated that the number of patients coming to the clinic daily had been between 100 and 160, but now had suddenly dropped to zero.[55]

Despite the uncompromising stance of both Western practitioners and cleric–healers towards 'hybrid' healers, the number of injectionists appears to have increased substantially from the 1940s through the 1970s, along with the proliferation of Western drugs and medical knowledge. This growth, while difficult to quantify, reflected a growing demand for medical practitioners to fill the gap created by the scarcity of Western medical facilities.

So where did the injectionists come from and how did they acquire their knowledge? Cleric–healers believed that a few crafty individuals, having some knowledge of botanical remedies, were the ones who first indulged in learning biomedical practices, notably prescribing antibiotics, with or without administering hypodermic injections, for their parents, relations or acquaintances.[56]

This view may be partially correct, but one can obtain a fuller view of their backgrounds from other written and oral sources. Though archival documents are almost silent about the ways in which the injectionists obtained their medical training in the 1950s and 1960s, there is some evidence that the injectionists constituted people who had some medical training and certification (as dressers or health assistants) and had served as full- or part-time injectionists in government clinics.[57] Only trained injectionists were properly instructed in how to administer injections. They were not taught how to contend with allergic or drug reactions of their treatments, nor were they entitled to diagnose illnesses or prescribe medicines.[58]

Interviews with current and former injectionists provide a richer picture of these pervasive purveyors of 'hybrid' medicine. These sources suggest that many injectionists received considerable training. A good number appear to have been retired individuals who had served as health assistants in the armed forces and public schools. One injectionist claimed to have been trained as a first-aid provider for an artillery unit. His training included how to take care of the wounded, including those with bone, joint and muscle injuries, and to arrest bleeding using a first-aid kit until a trained healthcare provider arrived. He claimed that some first-aid providers served as health assistants for trained medical practitioners who allowed them to receive additional training on how to observe the physical constitution of a patient so as to account for his or her sickness, including signs and symptoms of fever, diarrhoea, head or stomach aches, boils or lesions on the body or inflammation of the tonsils.

After some time, they also obtained instructions on how to use a stethoscope to listen to the breathing and heartbeat of patients, to take their pulse and to administer injections, along with some other commonly used medicinal prescriptions.[59]

In some ways, the training of injectionists resembled that of church–healers. Thus, an informant who had worked as an injectionist since the late 1950s observed: 'One had to be patient and obedient.' This meant establishing a relationship with a medical practitioner and spending years carefully listening to his words and watching him as he practised, before gaining enough knowledge to begin practising on his own. It had taken him nearly two years to master all the necessary knowledge. Describing his training, he remembered how '[a] physician slapped me on the face when I was about to give an injection to a patient without removing the air from the syringe as it should be.'[60] Through this training injectionists learnt how to prescribe medicines for different illnesses, how to administer antidotes and to avoid allergic or drug reactions. This was important knowledge, which the injectionists applied when they started practising medicine independently.

However, not all injectionists were trained. Several injectionists admitted to having joined the medical field without receiving formal training; they had simply learnt their skills from a trained injectionist who showed them how to administer injections. Initially, this group of injectionists had been employed in mission and public health facilities as guards, gardeners, cleaners or other similar low-status jobs. By establishing close relations with trained injectionists, these unskilled and preliterate workers were able to learn how to administer injections. However, the 'trainees' had very little opportunity to practise the techniques they observed. Thus, they were not allowed to give injections into arteries, muscles, veins or into or under the skin. What amounted to practical training was no more than observing closely when their mentors administered injections to their patients. After going through a long period of observation, at some point in time the 'trained' individuals would start injecting their own patients using a few reusable syringes.

While many injectionists learnt their skills in urban areas, their best opportunity for acquiring a clientele was to roam around in rural areas as itinerant injectionists.[61] Whatever the degree of their medical training, the injectionists as the embodiment of biomedicine, sold their utilitarian medical expertise to the rural public, including retailing medicines in their kiosks or drug shops.

The injectionists were able to dominate the market in the countryside, facing very little competition from government clinics situated in district capitals and along the main roads. To counter this situation, clinic administrators, relying on the support of local administrative officials, persistently tried to repress the injectionists. Ignoring the possibility that injectionists might actually play a role in supplementing the Western healthcare delivery system, clinic administrators frequently reminded sub-district governors to be vigilant of the injectionists working in their respective areas and to send patients directly to the government clinics.[62] Many government communications reported that injectionists and rural drug traders violated the law and posed potential health threats to local populations.[63] However, the fact of the matter was that the injectionists and drug traders competed effectively for biomedical clients in the rural areas. Biomedical institutions, in order to gain control of the medical marketplace, felt 'duty-bound' to take action against the injectionists.[64]

As long as the physical coverage of biomedical establishments remained restricted, the situation was hard to reverse. Though well aware of the limited nature of therapeutic options in rural settings, biomedical practitioners refused to acknowledge that injectionists and rural drug stores might have a role to play in the rural medical marketplace. They were more concerned with controlling the injectionists, whom they portrayed as exploiters of the preliterate public, than in rationalising the rural health system. Hence, the majority of clinic administrators persistently tried to tarnish the image of the injectionists.

In the face of these attacks, some injectionists sought to gain acceptance by applying for a work licence to serve as an injectionist.[65] The applicants stressed the need to create jobs so as to help themselves and their families.[66] Applications came not only from the places where there were no local health facilities, but also from a number of localities where government clinics had been functioning for years. These applications were not entertained, and health offices, as in the past, continued to point to the danger that could be created by unschooled practitioners who lacked even a modicum of elementary health education and whose medical knowledge was limited to giving injections.[67] Health workers also argued that untrained medical practitioners were damaging the reputation of biomedicine by mismanaging medication. Put differently, the 'unbridled action' of untrained practitioners and their pseudo-treatments were blamed for making the rural people less enthusiastic about Western medicine and for leading them to resort to village seers and other forms of indigenous medical treatment.[68]

To control the 'injectionists', who travelled from place to place with their syringes and tablets, clinic administrators sometimes requested the co-operation of the police. To do this, they linked injectionists to patient fatalities.[69] Some injectionists found themselves being repeatedly accused of causing harm to their patients.[70] Despite recurrent accusations against unlicensed practitioners, there was no effective mechanism to restrain them from their activities. The limited punishments provided for in the penal code did little to discourage repeated infringements by unlicensed healers.[71]

This situation did not show any sign of improvement in the early 1970s when, for example, an injectionist was accused of deceiving his patients by telling them that 'his injections and medicines were much better than similar products from the government clinics'. He was blamed for misinforming patients (while entertaining them with coffee) to accept his 'blessed' medicine.[72] The success of the injectionists in attracting clients through persuasion or deception may not be surprising in a province such as Wallo, where its estimated population of 3 million was served by three mission hospitals, a leprosarium, five health centres, twenty clinics,[73] and about 46 health workers (which amounted to one worker per 65 000 people) in 1967.[74] The only change that was visible in the province in 1971 was that the number of health centres and clinics had grown to eight and twenty-four respectively.[75] Yet even with this increase, four out of twelve districts had no health centres until 1973.[76]

The aggressive approach taken by health authorities towards the injectionists and other non-biomedical health practitioners did little to enhance the acceptance of Western medicine. At the same time, it deprived biomedical practitioners of the opportunity to learn how the injectionists popularised the injection needle in Ethiopian society. As a result, the information that could have been used to adapt Western medical practices to local cultural settings and develop accommodative or interventionist strategies was never collected.

Navigating the Medical Marketplace

In the end, efforts to eliminate competition from non-licensed providers of biomedical treatments failed and local populations continued to take advantage of the multiple sources of healing available in the Ethiopian medical marketplace. This should not be surprising. In many areas distance, transportation and treatment costs were serious problems, making the rural public's access to public health facilities almost impossible. This was especially true for people living in remote villages without government or mission-run healthcare facilities. These populations were left with two options: to suffer and die without getting any medical help or to look for and use other streams of alternative therapies.[77] Yet the decision to go to an injectionist or other provider of drugs was by no means obvious. A patient and his or her family were often faced with a number of therapeutic options and the decision to seek help from an injectionist often followed a lengthy set of deliberations.

As in other parts of Africa, illness sufferers played a negligible role in managing their own therapy. Families, neighbours, relatives and acquaintances played a crucial role in influencing patients' decisions. To help patients overcome their health problems, all these individuals made use of their intimate relationship with the patient and formed what Janzen called a 'therapy managing group'.[78] The group discussed the patient's condition and suggested possible lines of treatment based on their own experiences and opinions about different forms of therapy. These might include church healers, herbalists, application of holy water,[79] visiting an injectionist, obtaining tablets from a drug vendor, trying out a home-based remedy or visiting a government or mission-run clinic. Depending on the complexity of the case, the patient might be directed to employ more than one form of therapy.

More often than not, a cleric–diviner would be consulted before choosing a therapeutic course of action. Based on the diagnostic and therapeutic proposal of a cleric/spiritual healer–diviner, the patient's family would begin to act without delay, deciding where, how and when they should apply home-based remedies or obtain the recommended medicine from an indigenous healer. If this did not work out, a patient's family might consult another cleric/secular healer or shift their attention to a drug vendor or an injectionist. If this did not help, the final option was to take the patient to a nearby public health facility.

Those who chose to seek the aid of an injectionist did so for a number of reasons. In some cases local understandings of the aetiology or pathology of the disease indicated that it would be best treated by an injectionists; for example, the ideas surrounding an undifferentiated sickness called *mich* (a disease attributed to the influence of the sun, causing fever and aching of the whole body) often encouraged patients to seek treatment with hypodermic injections. The alleged therapeutic swiftness of injections in curing acute illnesses such as *mich*, a self-curing illness, prompted patients to attach particular importance to the hypodermic needle and the injectionists. The need for immediate relief from their illnesses made patients more enthusiastic about having injectable treatments than swallowing tablets for days. For most patients, the idea of taking tablets for a week or more was a serious problem. Those who acquiesced in biomedical treatment did not refrain from trying some home-based indigenous therapies such as drinking a herbal potion, rubbing the body with a concoction or inhaling the boiled steam of medicinal herbs.

In other cases, an injectionist was chosen for social reasons; for example, injectionists were often called on to treat patients with venereal disease, who, fearful of being censured or stigmatised, wished to avoid being treated at a public health clinic.[80] Many venereal disease patients, who wanted to conceal or were unwilling to admit to having sexually transmitted diseases, did not immediately come to the injectionists because it was widely believed that to have an injection would only bring short-term relief and not result in a lasting cure; hence, the saying, መርፌ አትወጉ በሽታውን ይደብቀዋል ('Do not take an injection because it hides away the disease').

There were also reasons why a patient might avoid an injectionist; for example, it was believed that diseases caused by the action of certain spirits might be made worse by an injection. This was because the needle could hurt the disease-causing spirit, causing it to endanger the life of the patient by making him or her unresponsive to other therapeutic or exorcising procedures.

Having decided to send a patient to an injectionist, a patient's management group would look for someone who enjoyed unquestionable skill and reputation. The adage እጁ መድኃኒት ነው (‘He has a curing hand’ or ‘His hand is medicinal’) expressed the need for an injectionist with a reputation for bringing immediate relief and for administering injections without hurting his patients. An additional characteristic looked for in an injectionist was his comforting gesture and ability to instil a spirit of encouragement into his troubled clients. Injectionists did more than inject medicines into their clients. They also offered advice on how to manage diseases, through controlling diet, avoiding too much worrying and on the value of being emotionally strong. The ability to manage sickness was as important as the ability to inject medicines.[81]

Moreover, in some cases the injectionists would even refuse to give an injection to a seriously ill patient, fearing that he might be held accountable for the patient's death; a situation that could readily be exploited by the health authorities. It was not uncommon for a patient's death to be attributed to incorrect medication being administered by an injectionist. In other cases, injectionists discouraged patients from going for treatments with an injection needle because they felt that some other form of therapy, such as inhaling the boiling steam of a concoction of medicinal herbs or drawing blood through bloodletting or spiritual treatments, would be more effective.[82]

More often than not, however, patients visiting an injectionist expected to receive injectable treatments. As one injectionist aptly put it: ‘With the exception of a few ailments that can easily be distinguished by looking at the condition of patients, the best therapeutic choice for almost all human maladies was the injection needle.’[83] Informants believed that they administered injections in response to the demands of their clients. Many patients came with the preconceived assumption of getting immediate relief from their sickness with injectable medicines; and it was not an easy undertaking, underlined an injectionist, ‘to persuade patients not to have injection or to try other treatment modalities’.[84] To satisfy the wishes of inflexible clients, at times the injectionists resorted to administering distilled water to their patients. This action, which was based on absolute trust in injectionists, may have assisted in weakening the hold of a disease on a patient and speeded up his or her recovery. This treatment method, which had some placebo effect, 'had more to do with psychological than with real biological or therapeutic worth,'[85] reasoned an informant.

Even when the treatment of choice was the injection, injectionists would be mindful of advising in accordance with their patients' socially rooted perceptions and understandings of the causes of their sickness. In this regard, they differed in a fundamental way from biomedical practitioners who refused to acknowledge the importance of these understandings; for example, the injectionists advised gonorrhoea-afflicted individuals, whom they injected with penicillin, to avoid exposure to the sun while urinating or not to urinate on the spot where a dog had previously urinated. Both actions were believed to cause sexually transmitted diseases.[86] After giving injections, they also questioned patients with a venereal disease about their spouse, suggesting that they encouraged patients to abstain from sexual contacts for some time, and to persuade and bring their wives to have similar treatments.

In order to boost the efficacy of their treatments and to maintain their reputation, injectionists offered advice to their patients; for instance, they advised patients to wash their bodies and maintain their personal hygiene; to have adequate rest; to prevent constipation and to go to the restroom on a regular basis; to clean their teeth with brushing sticks; and to take hot drinks or foods. Many injectionists also forbade patients from taking salty, fatty or highly fermented foods, coffee and local beverages with strong alcoholic contents, and engaging in licentious sexual behaviours.[87]

Providing treatment at patients' homes was one of the acclaimed services of the injectionists. They went to the homes of the sick to provide emergency medical assistance, to help pregnant women deliver their babies[88] or to give them injections. They gave injections either early in the morning or after sunset; the two most preferred times to administer injections. The idea of giving injections during these times of the day was to keep patients away from the evil influence of the midday sun, which was believed to aggravate many illness conditions. Occasionally, injectionists helped their patients to procure prescribed medicines from pharmacies; and they encouraged the sick to eat some food before receiving treatment, to lie down when given injections and to drink water after treatments had been administered.

While injectionists and drug dealers were the primary means by which many Ethiopians accessed elements of Western biomedicine, they were not the only ones to incorporate Western biomedical ideas and practices into their treatment; in fact, some literate cleric– and herbalist–healers were in the habit of consulting biomedical texts originally written in Amharic or, in most cases, texts translated from English as medical handbooks.[89] They applied this textually oriented knowledge in identifying or diagnosing and treating a range of illnesses.[90]

The majority of cleric–healers rebuffed the unmethodical use of biomedical products. 'We always condemned the mixing of biomedical and indigenous medicaments, and had very little doubt regarding the questionable personality and medical training of those who engaged in this kind of activity,'[91] underscored one informant. They also asked: 'How could a person with no Western education and biomedical training dare to prescribe or include, openly or secretly, products of biomedicine in his treatment regimen?' For most informants, the move by some practitioners away from conventional practices was tantamount to collaborating with those who would want to undermine the reputation of ingenuous healers.

However, the majority of secular healers (and a few cleric–healers too) supported the idea of utilising some tools of biomedicine, such as gloves, scissors, plaster and bandages. These tools were valuable in treating open wounds, and rendering efficient and hygienic medical services, they argued. They also acknowledged the importance of referring patients to Western medical institutions when faced with health problems that lay beyond their ability.[92]

The increasing influence of Western allopathic medicine can be detected from the healers' lists of disease names. To attract clients, many cleric–healers publicised in their advertisement posters illnesses such as amoeba, jardiasis, gastritis, typhoid, tuberculosis, bronchitis, asthmatics, diabetics, epilepsy, blood pressure and cancer (disease names almost entirely unknown in indigenous medical texts). It appears that accessing the few translated biomedical texts, which began to appear since the mid-twentieth century, gave literate cleric–healers the opportunity to acquaint themselves with Western labels for illnesses. Previously, many illnesses known by a generic term such as *colic*, *dysentery* or *cough* were simply identified with specific parts of the human body, such as abdomen and chest.[93] The adoption of Western illness labels also modified some disease aetiologies, expanding ideas of causation that had emphasised the role of external spirits to include internal physiological processes.

Employing biomedical aetiologies and nomenclatures did not signify a deviation from the traditional diagnostic methods, nor did it herald the discovery of new drug plants and/or the perfection of healers' treatments. Most healers continued to use 'old' medicines recommended in the local medical texts;[94] for instance, tuberculosis and asthma being diagnosed as 'chest diseases' were commonly treated with indigenous medications recommended for chronic coughing. Many abdominal problems, albeit symptomatically diagnosed, were also treated with the medicines commonly prescribed in local medical texts. For the mentally disturbed, indigenous healers utilised the few prosaic medicines customarily used to treat patients' allegedly ensorcelled or attacked by evil-eyed people, noxious spirits or magic spells known commonly as *buda*, *aynatila*, *likift*[95] or *digimt*.[96]

In the end, cleric–healers had only the vaguest understanding of the biomedical aetiologies of the new disease categories they adopted.[97] It is likely that, to a large degree, their replacement of indigenous labels for illnesses with biomedical ones represented a marketing strategy aimed at attracting clients from a population that was becoming increasingly familiar with biomedical categories. It was, in other words, a means of maintaining their claim to a share of an increasingly competitive medical marketplace.

Conclusion

Replacing 'unorthodox' medical practices with conventional biomedicine proved impossible during the imperial period. Lack of biomedical resources, particularly in the rural areas, combined with bureaucratic inefficiencies, meant that Western-style medical care was difficult to access and public health interventions had limited impact on the health of the Ethiopian population. In addition, practitioners of biomedicine made little effort to understand indigenous medical concepts and practices, and to develop approaches to health care, which build on these understandings. It is, therefore, hardly surprising that alternative forms of therapy were widely used.

While government health authorities often decried these practices, they had little to offer that would encourage patients to abandon them. This did not mean, however, that the Ethiopian public had no contact with elements of Western biomedicine. Many patients received injections, and consumed antibiotics and other Western pharmaceuticals. However, a growing army of illegal injectionists and drug shops provided these services, not the government and missionary medical establishments. Likewise, other secular healers, and to a lesser degree cleric–healers, integrated certain biomedical ideas, technologies and terminologies into their medical practice, while maintaining older ideas about disease causation and cure, in order to compete in the urban medical marketplace. The popularity of these various 'hybrid' therapies lay in their ability to bridge the conceptual divide between Western biomedicine and indigenous belief systems.

The health situation of the majority of the rural masses, who lived 'on the borderline' between the two medical worlds, was not substantially changed even after the overthrow of the imperial regime in the early 1970s. This situation confirmed that the transformation to an era of modern scientific medicine was indefinitely postponed. It also proved that a substantial increase in the healthcare coverage of the people with the costly, technologically based scientific medicine remained a distant dream. As long as the curative services of allopathic medicine remained more distant and inefficient, indigenous medicine being readily available was 'increasingly appreciated'.[98] In such a situation, to endorse and promote a pluralistic medical system may have been a viable option.

Figure 13: A typical magic scroll

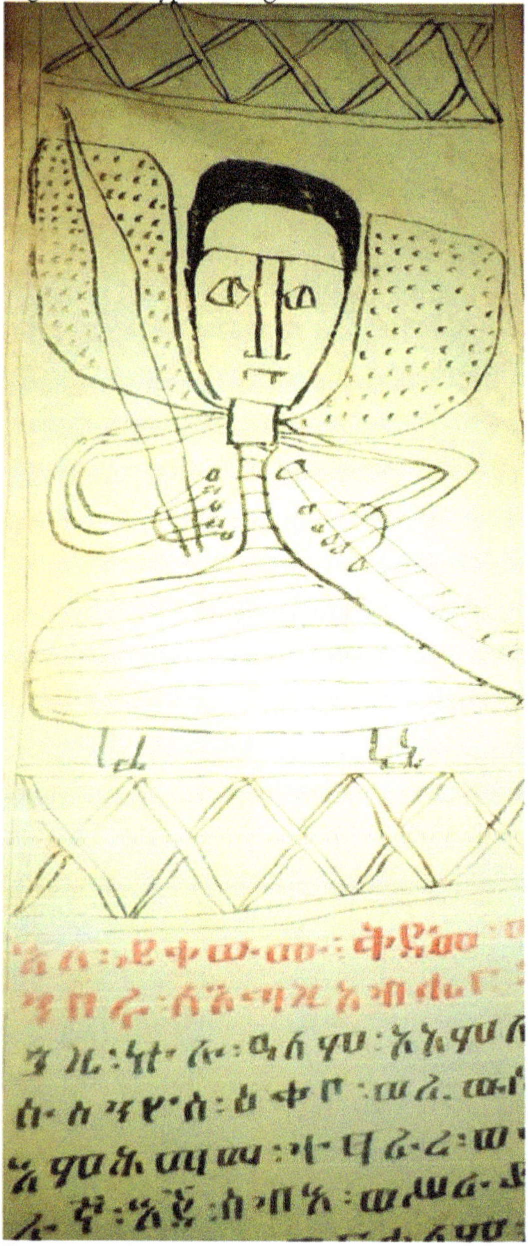

Source: IES Ms. No. 5561:

Figure 14: A protective amulet written for a certain Wolde Yohannes

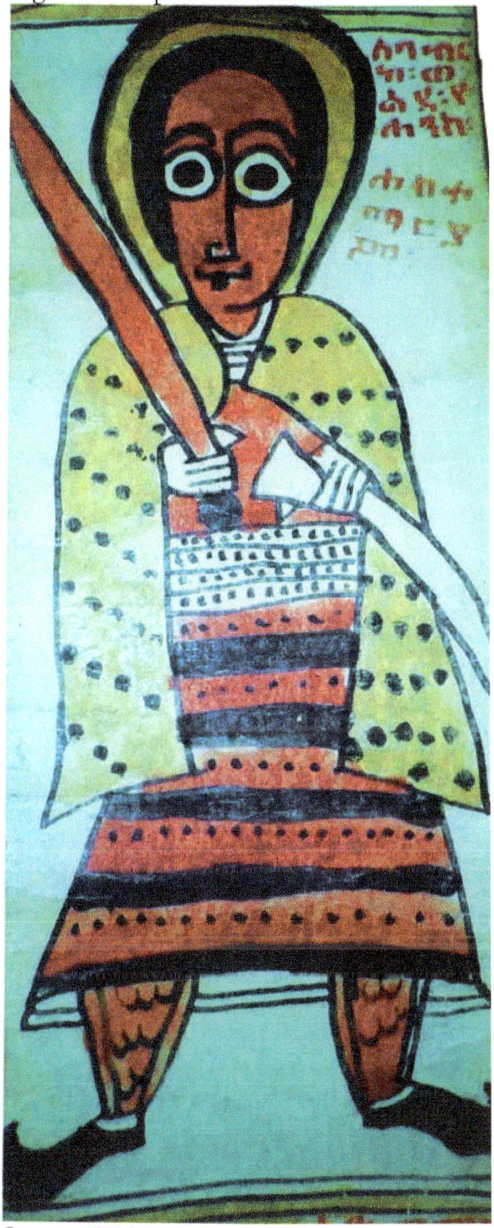

Source: IES Ms. No. 5561b

Figure 15: An image to ensnare the devil

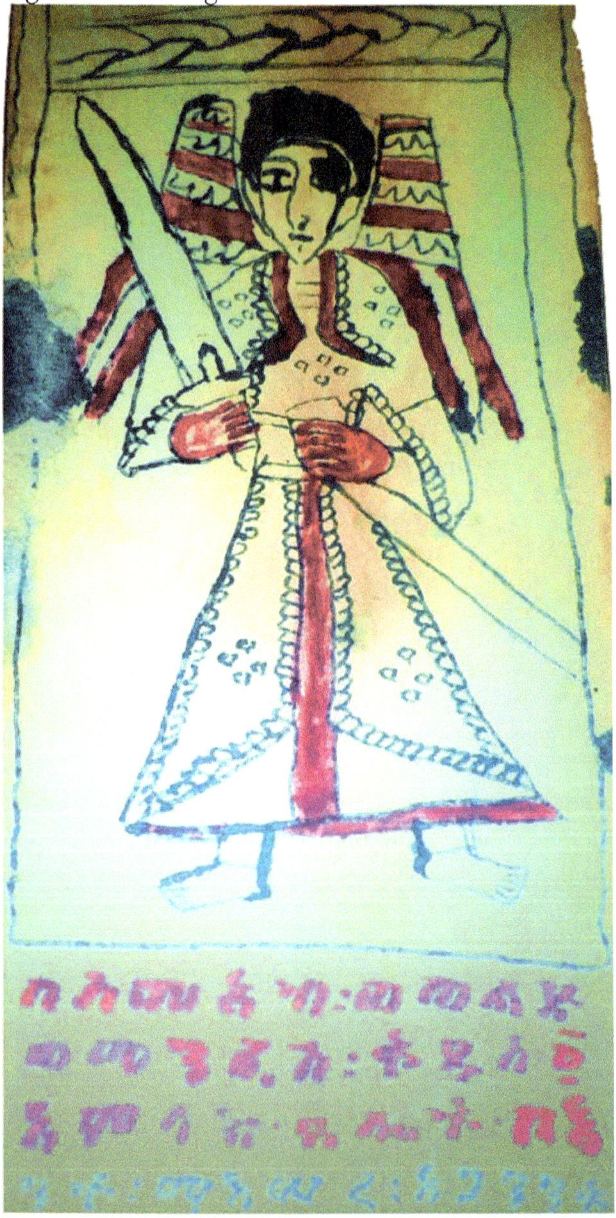

Source: IES Ms. No. 4448

Notes

1 Both Janzen and Good have described the range of therapeutic options available to the Zairian and Kenyan public. In Zaire (now the Democratic Republic of Congo), Janzen argued, no therapeutic institution or practitioner dominated the healing profession whereby the sufferers and their advocates, whom he called 'therapy managing group', took every opportunity to make therapeutic choices from among herbalists, magicians, biomedical practitioners and prophet diviners. Though indigenous and Western medicine coexisted at every level of Zairian society, Janzen made it clear that Western medicine was trusted only 'over a limited range of physical symptoms and signs'. Good's findings confirmed the significant role played by indigenous medical practitioners and their therapies, though catering principally for the rural public, had considerable influence on the lives of the urban dwellers. John Janzen, *The Quest for Therapy in Lower Zaire* (Berkeley: University of California, 1978), 221 225. Charles Good, *Ethnomedical Systems in Africa: Patterns of Traditional Medicine in Rural and Urban Kenya* (New York: Guilford Press, 1978a).

2 Paul Henze, 'Movement Towards Modernization: A Century of Progress', in *The Ecology of Health and Disease in Ethiopia*, edited by Helmut Kloos and Zein Ahmed Zein (Colorado: Westview Press, 1993), 12.

3 See Ministry of Interior, file no. 4/2; G. G. Campbell, Director General of Medical Services, 'Memorandum for the U.N.R.R.A. Mission to Ethiopia,' 11 February 1946; the memorandum talks about the country's need for substantial quantities of vaccines and dichlorodiphenyltrichloroethane (DDT) to combat epidemic typhus, of which several rare types were said to be spreading.

4 Italian-built roads and communications played a pivotal role in the government's effort to reunify the country.

5 Workneh Kassie and Helmut Kloos, 'Modern Health Services', in *The Ecology of Health and Disease in Ethiopia*, 135; see also Asrat Waldayes, 'The Postliberation Period (1941–1973),' in *An Introduction to the Medical History of Ethiopia*, edited by Richard Pankhurst (Trenton, NJ: The Red Sea Press, 1990), 246–248.

6 With the exception of the Mikitil Woredas, which was abolished in 1973, this administrative structure was maintained until the mid-1980s. Dessalegn Rahmato, *The Peasant and the State: Studies in Agrarian Change in Ethiopia, 1950s–2000s* (Addis Ababa: Addis Ababa University Press, 2009), 115; see also Asmelash Beyene, 'Some Notes on the Evolution

of Regional Administration in Ethiopia,' *Ethiopian Journal of Development Research*, 9(1) (1987): 37, 40–41.

7 Dessalegn Rahmato, *The Peasant and the State*, 115. For a meticulous discussion on the administrative structure of the imperial regime, see John Markakis, *Ethiopia: Anatomy of a Traditional Polity* (Oxford: Oxford University Press, 1974), 288ff.

8 Ibid., 313.

9 At times, requests were sent to the emperor before any action was taken. Ministry of Interior, file no. 131, Crown Prince Asfa Wossen to Haile Selassie (telegram), 23 May 1945.

10 Ministry of Interior, file no. 41. Ministry of Health to the Gojjam Hospital, 27 September 1952.

11 Ministry of Interior, file no. 37/50. Wallo Provincial Clinic Administration to Wallo Provincial Governorate Office, 14 January 1946. It is worth noting that the former Wallo Provincial Clinic Administration Office was to become Wallo Provincial Public Health Office in 1963. See Dessie Hospital, file no. ኢ-22.

12 Eyassu Habte-Gabr, 'Typhus and Other Rickettsial Diseases,' in *the Ecology of Health and Disease in Ethiopia.* 411; even in the 1980s, noted Eyassu, incidents of typhus fever were diagnosed 'as cases of acute febrile illness [and treated] with commonly used antibiotics'. Ibid.

13 Dessie Municipality, file no. መ3-5. Ministry of Health to Wallo Provincial Governorate Office, n.d. Those who had been vaccinated against typhus routinely complained about reinfection with the same disease. These individuals were actually suffering from relapsing fever, an illness with no preventative vaccine. Many typhus-vaccinated individuals, thinking that their immunity from typhus would also protect them from symptomatically similar maladies, did not refrain from mingling with people infected with relapsing fever. Lack of knowledge of what epidemiologists referred to as 'agent–host–environment chain' was the main reason why typhus-immunised people considered anti-typhoid vaccine as 'pure water, not a potent medicine'.

14 Ministry of Interior, file no. 131-መ 5. Ministry of Health to Wallo Provincial Governorate Office, 5 October 1966.

15 See Mesfin Wolde Mariam, *Rural Vulnerability to Famine in Ethiopia: 1958–1977* (New Delhi: Vikas Publishing House, 1984), 105.

16 Wallo Provincial Health Department, file no. ጲ-17, 23 May 1966.

17 Mesfin Wolde Mariam, *Rural Vulnerability to Famine in Ethiopia*, 10.

18 Ministry of Interior, file no. 131-መ 5, Epidemiology Department to the Wallo Provincial Governorate Office, 9 September 1958.

19 Ibid.

20 This specialised unit began its work in the early 1950s, along with smallpox and malaria eradication units.

21 Wallo Provincial Health Department, file no. ደ-17, Wallo Provincial Governorate Office to Ministry of Interior, 6 June 1959; Wallo Provincial Governorate Office to the Ministry of Health, 10 June 1959. It is worth noting that the first three health centres were established in 1961, including the one in Dessie. Ministry of Public Health, 'Directory of Medical and Health Institutions in Ethiopia' (Addis Ababa: January 1972), 14.

22 Ministry of Interior, file no. 4/2. The Health Department in the Ministry of Interior to the Ministry of Interior, 29 April 1946.

23 Ibid; similar issues were raised in the 1960s, see, for example, Wallo Regional Ministry of Health, file no. ደ-17, Asfa Wossen Hospital to Dessie Zuria District Governorate Office, March 22, 1964.

24 Ministry of Interior, file no. 22/22, Begemdir and Semen Provincial Governorate Office to the Ministry of Interior Health Department, 25 April 1946.

25 Wallo Provincial Health Department, file no. ደ-17. Debebe Tadege, 'Epidemic Report', 29 October 1965.

26 Ministry of Interior, file no. 41. Ministry of Health to the Gojjam Provincial Governorate Office, n.d.

27 John Markakis, *Ethiopia: Anatomy of a Traditional Polity*, 291.

28 Ministry of Interior, file no. 41, Ministry of Health to the Ministry of Interior, 22 March 1962.

29 Ibid.

30 Asrat Waldayes, 'The Postliberation Period (1941–1973)', in Richard Pankhurst, *An Introduction to the Medical History of Ethiopia*, 248, 263.

31 Ministry of Interior, file no. 131-መ5, Malaria Eradication Service to the Provincial Governor of Wallo, 29 February 1967; Ministry of Interior, file no. 143-መ5, Kidane Alemu to the Wallo Provincial Department of Health, August 1967.

32 Ministry of Interior, file no. 143-መ5, Kidane Alemu to the Wallo Provincial Department of Health, 24 September 1967.

33 Ministry of Interior, file no. መ 5/27, Ministry of Health to the Ministry of Interior, 14 July 1956.

34 Richard Pankhurst, *An Introduction to the Medical History of Ethiopia*, 26–28.

35 Ministry of Interior, file no. 131-መ5, Governor of Wallo Province to the Minister of Health, 22 March 1969. The governor also wrote about the refusal of the people to allow medical treatment in the hands of the two women physicians working in the provincial hospital. Ibid., 22 July 1968.

36 Ministry of Interior, file no. 131-መ5, Wallo Provincial Governorate Office to the Ministry of Health, 24 March 1965.

37 Order no. 22 of 1960, 'An Order to Provide for the Administration of the Health Tax'. A similar edict had been promulgated in the late 1940s as Proclamation no. 91 of 1947.

38 Likewise, the provincial governors presiding over the Provincial Advisory Health Councils were theoretically empowered to administer health taxes, that is, to expand and improve 'public health facilities in their respective provinces.' Ibid. See also Ministry of Interior, file no. 41. Ministry of Interior to the 13 Provincial and 2 District Governorate Offices, 8 November 1960.

39 Hospitals such as Bethesda (established in the 1920s and renamed later *Haile Selassie I Hospital*), St Paul (established in the 1940s and initially administered under the Ministry of Health) and Gandhi (a maternity hospital founded in the 1950s with the help of the Indian community) in Addis Ababa, and that of Ras Mekonnen hospital in Harar were among the few health institutions allegedly catering for the poor. See, *Haile Selassie I Foundation: 1945–1965* (Amharic) (Addis Ababa: Berhanena Selam Printing Press, 1965 E.C.); also Abera Jemberre, *Establishment of the Haile Selassie I Foundation.* (Amharic) (Addis Ababa: Berhanena Selam Printing Press, 1952 E.C.).

40 Medical personnel from the armed forces and government schools were sometimes accused of private medical practices. Wallo Provincial Health Department, file no. ወ-6, Hayq District Clinic to Ambassel District Governorate Office, 26 June 1959.

41 Though private medical practice was discouraged, the Ministry of Health was either less strict about or unable to prevent 'many national and expatriate doctors [from] indulg[ing] in office-clinics, for a small number of hours, outside their working day'. Asrat Waldayes, 'The Postliberation Period (1941–1973)', in *An Introduction to the Medical History of Ethiopia*, edited by Richard Pankhurst, 250.

42 The letter arguing in a populist tone goes on to say that 'the conflict that has come about because of private interest should not be permitted to further diminish the quality and extent of the medical practitioner's [sic] services nor should it interfere with the medical practitioners' duty to study and keep themselves abreast of new developments in medicine so that they may render better services to their patients.' Ministry of Interior, file no. 41, The Minister of Health, Circular, July 1964.

43 Ibid.

44 Wallo Provincial Health Department, file no. ደ-17, Ministry of Health to Teferi Mekonnen Adventist Mission Hospital and the Sudan Interior

Mission Hospital, telegrams nos. 104, 105, 106, 107, October, 1958, Ministry of Health to Teferi Mekonnen Hospital, 8 December 1958.

45 See David Talbot, *Haile Selassie I: Silver Jubilee* (The Hague: W. P. Van Stockum & Zoon, 1955), 265.

46 Wallo Provincial Health Department, file no. ወ-6, Teferi Yimer to Wallo Provincial Health Department, 11 June 1974.

47 Simon Messing, 'The Highland Plateau Amhara of Ethiopia,' unpublished PhD dissertation (University of Pennsylvania, 1957), 579–696.

48 Dawit Abebe and Ahadu Ayehu, *Medicinal Plants and Enigmatic Health Practices of Northern Ethiopia.* (Addis Ababa: Berhanena Salam Printing Press, 1993), 3.

49 This principle may also apply to indigenous healing where some illnesses may not have been properly understood or dealt with if patients had been denied the opportunity to discuss their problems openly with indigenous healers.

50 G. M. Foster, 'An Introduction to Ethnomedicine', In *Traditional Medicine and Health care Coverage*, edited by R. H. Bannermann, J, Burton and W. C. Chen (Geneva: World Health Organization, 1983), 17–24.

51 For a passing remark on the expansion of Western medicine and the 'emergence of a new and growing number of pseudo-modern "injectionists"', see Mekonnen Bishaw, 'Promoting Traditional Medicine in Ethiopia,' *Social Science and Medicine*, 33(2) (1991): 195; Slikkerveer called the injectionists 'specialists' of the transitional medical system; see Leendert Slikkerveer, 'Rural Health Development in Ethiopia: Problems of Utilization of Traditional Healers,' *Social Science and Medicine*, 16 (1982): 1863.

52 Oral informants nos. 1, 2, 5, 9 and 23.

53 Wallo Provincial Health Department, file no. ዴ-17, Mohammed Wolde to Wallo Provincial Health Department, 31 September 1966.

54 Wallo Provincial Health Department, file no. ወ-6, Gobena Yimer to Wallo Provincial Health Department, 24 July 1971.

55 Ibid.

56 Ibid.

57 Wallo Provincial Health Department, file no. ወ-6, Hayq District Clinic to Ambassel District Governorate Office, 26 June 1959.

58 Wallo Provincial Health Department, file no. ወ-6, Asfa Wossen Hospital to Wallo Provincial Police, 6 January 1958; for the persistence of this problem, see Wallo Provincial Health Department, file no. ወ-6, Wallo Provincial Governorate Office to the 12 District Governorate Offices, 2 July 1972.

59 Oral informant no. 61.

60 Ibid. After quitting his military career he went back to his rural village and began to serve as an 'injectionist'. He later moved to a provincial town and continued his medical career until he stopped due to ill-health almost a year later.

61 Oral informants nos. 61, 62 and 63.

62 Wallo Provincial Health Department, file no. ወ-6, Hayq District Clinic to Ambassel District Governorate Office, 26 June 1959; Wallo Provincial Health Department to Borena District Governorate Office, 23 August 1963; Wallo Provincial Health Department, file no. ወ-6, Wallo Provincial Health Department to Sayo Tebela Sub-District Governorate Office, 27 September 1962.

63 Referring to the more than half-a-dozen letters written to the provincial hospital in the period between 1950 and 1960, the head of a government clinic complained about the lack of legal measures being taken against unlicensed drug shops in its district; see Wallo Provincial Health Department, file no. ወ-6, Qallu District Clinic to Asfa Wossen Hospital, 8 June 1960.

64 Wallo Provincial Health Department, file no. ወ-6, Raya and Kobo District Clinic to the Ministry of Health, 19 May 1959; Wallo Provincial Governorate Office to the Twelve District Governorate Offices, 2 July 1970.

65 Wallo Provincial Health Department, file no. ወ-6, Wallo Provincial Health Department to Sayo Tebela Sub-district Governorate Office, 27 September 1962.

66 Ibid.

67 Wallo Provincial Health Department, file no. ወ-6, Gebre Medhin Gebre Egzi to Wallo Provincial Department of Health, 8 March 1971; Wallo Provincial Department of Health to the Borena District Governorate Office, 23 August 1963; Wag District Clinic to Wag District Police, 7 November 1959; Hayq District Clinic to Ambassel District Governorate Office, 26 June 1959; Qallu District Clinic to Asfa Wossen Hospital, 8 June 1959; Raya and Kobo District Clinic to the Ministry of Health, 19 May 1959; Asfa Wossen Hospital to the Wallo Provincial Police, 7 March 1959; Wallo Provincial Health Department to the Wallo Provincial Governorate Office, 12 May 1971.

68 Wallo Provincial Health Department, file no. ወ-6, Gebre Medhin Gebre Egzi to Wallo Provincial Governorate Office, 8 April 1971.

69 Wallo Provincial Health Department, file no. ወ-6, Wallo Provincial Governorate Office to the Twelve District Governorate Offices, 2 July 1970. Article 518 entitled 'unlawful exercises of the medical or public health professions' was applicable to offenders. See Penal Code 1957.

70 Wallo Provincial Health Department, file no. ወ-6, Asfa Wossen Hospital to the Wallo Provincial Police, 7 March 1959.

71 'Whosoever, having neither the professional qualifications prescribed and controlled by the competent authority nor the authorisation to set up in official practice . . . is punishable with simple imprisonment and fine.' See the 1957 Ethiopian Penal Code, Art. 518(1).

72 Wallo Provincial Health Department, file no. ወ-6, Asfa Wossen Hospital to the Wallo Provincial Police, 7 March 1959.

73 Wen-Pin Chang, 'Development of Basic Health Services in Ethiopia.' Reprinted from the *Journal of the Formosan Medical Association*, 68(6) (1969): 309. The first three health centres, including the one in Dessie, were established in 1961. See Ministry of Public Health, 'Directory of Medical and Health Institutions in Ethiopia', January 1972, 14; during 1960–1965, the period of the First Five-Year Plan, the number of health centres at a national level was no more than 58.

74 Dessie Hospital, file no. 32/ኮ10/2, 17 June 1966.

75 Ministry of Public Health, 'Directory of Medical and Health Institutions in Ethiopia,' January 1972, 8.

76 The number of doctors in Ethiopia in 1973 was about 370, of which the great majority were expatriate, and of whom about 70 per cent were working in major towns such as Addis Ababa, Asmara and Harar. See Richard Pankhurst, *An Introduction to the Medical History of Ethiopia*, 263.

77 In predominantly Muslim communities, preparing *wadaja* ritual (a specialised session for group prayers) was one of the easiest options. The *wadaja* seemed compulsory when a community was affected by communicable diseases (human or animal), and natural calamities such as drought, heavy rain and locust invasion. The ritual was also used for healing purposes when, for example, the family of the sick would summon *wadaja* experts to conduct a healing session to free the sick from physical or socio-psychological illness and help the patient regain his/her health. It is worth noting that the role of the *wadaja* in indigenous healing is an important area of serious investigation.

78 John Janzen, *The Quest for Therapy in Lower Zaire*, 224–225.

79 When families had a hard time deciding on a particular holy water, for example, they prepared rolled pieces of paper in which names of holy waters were written and asked the patient to draw one of the papers randomly.

80 For 'injectionists', offering such a discreet service was an important means of establishing strong social networks and obtaining gifts from their clients and former patients.

81 Asrat Waldayes, 'The Postliberation Period (1941–1973)', in *An Introduction to the Medical History of Ethiopia,* edited by Richard Pankhurst,

245. Abstinence from spicy or peppery foods and alcoholic drinks was part of their treatment regimen; this idea was reminiscent of the Italian period.

82 They recommended bloodletting for undifferentiated febrile illnesses and spiritual treatments for some psycho-social or mental illnesses.

83 Oral informant no. 61.

84 Ibid.

85 Oral informant no. 62.

86 To avoid contracting haemorrhoids, they advised their clients not to sit on a hot spot or not to relieve themselves at or near the spot where a person with haemorrhoids had previously relieved himself or herself. They also advised that a person took care not to get sick from contaminated water, malnourishment, and abuse of alcohol and bites of certain insects.

87 Oral informants nos. 61, 62 and 63; the injectionists strongly believed that to lead a healthy life a person had to eat different kinds of diets, and not to do so could expose him or her to a variety of ailments. They also considered some foods potential sources of ill-health.

88 A few injectionists were also skilled in removing troubling teeth.

89 A good example of this is a popular medical handbook entitled *Yatena Mogzit* (Guardian of Health) translated into Amharic and published in 1958 E.C. It is noted in the preface that '[s]ince the last ten years biomedicine has made great strides in offering curative services to hundreds of thousands of people, which was not the case before a decade. Now the publication of this medical text would help many people understand the causes of many illnesses and treat themselves.' Hubert Swartut, *Yatena Mogzit (Guardian of Health)*,trans. Abebe Bezuneh (Addis Ababa: Adventist Printing Press, 1966).

90 Oral informant no. 30.

91 Oral informants nos. 2, 26, 29 and 37.

92 Oral informants nos. 6, 11, 23, 27, 35, 37 and 52.

93 As Young put it, healers' physiological notions 'are simple [and] they do not link etiologies to syndromes in a highly differentiated way . . . [while] in the abstract each etiology is linked to a typical syndrome.' Allan Young, 'Externalizing and Internalizing Medical Beliefs: An Ethiopian Example', *Social Science and Medicine*, 10 (3/4) (1976): 150.

94 Ibid.

95 *Likift* was commonly used to designate illnesses that attacked the skin (e.g., leprosy, scabies and eczema) and other animal–human contagions. *Likift* was mostly contracted by ingesting or washing with water previously touched, tasted or breathed upon by demons. Even leprosy,

the most feared disease, was the result of contagion with demon-infested water.

96 Oral informant no. 30.

97 Oral informants nos. 6, 11, 23, 27, 35, 37 and 52; posting advertisements in newspapers and magazines became a common scene after the overthrow of the Darg in 1991. Before that, indigenous healers used to post lists of illnesses side by side with the medicaments that were meant to be sold in the markets and along the main roads.

98 Asrat Waldayes, 'The Postliberation Period (1941–1973),' in *An Introduction to the Medical History of Ethiopia*, edited by Richard Pankhurst, 253.

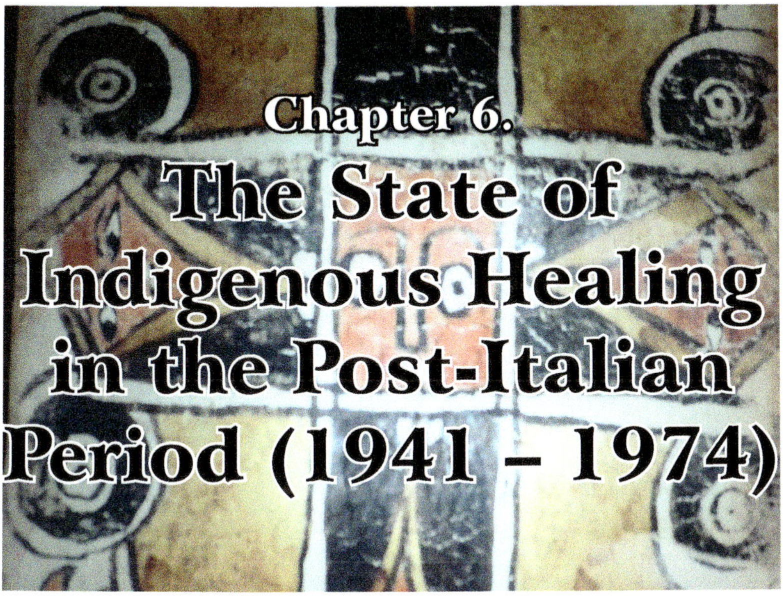

Chapter 6. The State of Indigenous Healing in the Post-Italian Period (1941 – 1974)

The chapter examines the position of cleric–healers during the imperial era. It focuses on how the state's efforts to legalise indigenous medicine supported state structures to limit the ability of church-based healers to function freely. The inability of Western biomedical services to meet the growing health needs of the Ethiopian population during the post-Italian period provided opportunities for a range of alternative therapies to compete for clients. These included the so called injectionists and others who combined biomedicine with indigenous medical ideas and practices, and older forms of healing, including those provided by clerical healers. While health officials in the new imperial government attempted to suppress hybrid therapists, whom they viewed as challenging the credibility of Western biomedicine, they adopted a more accommodative attitude towards indigenous healers; in fact, it was widely believed during the imperial period that indigenous healers penetrated Ethiopian society ranging from the imperial court[1] to the lowest level of government offices and ordinary households.[2]

Cleric-healers During the Imperial Era

In contrast to the Italian efforts to suppress indigenous healers, the restored imperial government tried to accommodate them in Ethiopia's medical system through a system of registration. While this permitted church-based healers to practise openly, their ability to do so was limited by the continued exercise of the discretionary authority of local officials, who had the power to limit or encourage such activities. At the same time, the position of church-based healers was challenged by other forms of healing and particularly by the growing popularity of spiritual healers. These spiritual healers, known sometimes as *qallicha*, not only competed directly for clients in the medical marketplace, they also engaged in activities that government authorities viewed as threats to state security. Government efforts to limit the activities of these spiritual healers negatively affected the lives of church-based healers, whose medical practices were sometimes confused with those of spiritual healers. In the end, the imperial era brought opportunities and challenges to church-based healers.

It was widely believed that Haile Selassie's power was augmented by the knowledge and wisdom provided by a host of cleric–diviners and hermit–monks.[3] Multiple stories about the emperor stressed this connection. One such story claimed that Qorit, a powerful demon with one leg, helped high officials of the imperial regime. According to the tale, Qorit had dwelled in a crater lake at the peak of mount Zeqwala, near Addis Ababa. However, Qorit had been driven away to another lake (Bishaftu) by Gabra Manfas Qedus to whom the Ethiopian Orthodox Church had dedicated the fifth day of each month. The venerated saint subsequently erected the famous Abbo Monastery beside the lake. The father of one of the emperor's ministers was a priest associated with this monastery. He is said to have acquired the magical formula to 'tame' Qorit and given it to his son.[4] This formula also allowed the emperor to harness Qorit's power and use it for his own ends. The alleged importance of Qorit's power for the emperor is said to explain the emperor's frequent visits to the demon's home at Lake Bishaftu.[5]

It is also said that a number of hermit monks, including a famous diviner–monk residing at Saint Gabriel Church, close to the imperial court, used to send prophesies to the emperor on a regular basis;[6] and near the close of Haile Selassie's era, several Orthodox and Muslim diviners and oracles were said to have sent their prophesies[7] or requested to meet the emperor in person.[8]

The links between cleric–healers and other administration officials are said to have been pervasive. Cleric–healers provided the privileged classes, notably government authorities and their families, with different kinds of protective amulets and fortune-bearing charms, such as ቅብአተ መንግስት ወሲመት፡ ፍቅረ መኳንንት ወፍቅረ ሕዝብ አሕዛብ ፡ ፀሎት በእንተ ሢመት ወቅብአት[9] (prayer(s) to obtain appointment and grace from the state, and prayer(s) to get the affection of dignitaries and the public). This suggested that the elite classes seeking to retain or advance their socio-economic and political positions were among the principal consumers of the magico-medical expertise of the literate cleric–healers.[10]

It was also not unusual for local governors and the landed gentry to send their messengers to cleric–healers and celibate diviners living in retreat in monasteries to obtain information on the auspiciousness of the year, outbreak of epidemic disease(s), famine and the stability or security of the state.[11] Diviners were the 'obvious experts to consult' on a range of personal or communal issues.

Cleric–healers also aided litigants seeking to win court cases. Litigation on issues concerning rural agricultural lands and inheritances was extensive during the imperial era, and litigants did what they could to influence the rulings of court judges using specially prepared magical prayers or *abinet*.[12] Many litigants seeking to prevail over their opponents were known to have consulted cleric–healers in the hope of getting their cases favourably heard by court judges. The clerics, in turn, acquired influence with magistrates by providing them with services.

Cleric–healers also dispensed education *abinet* to local authorities and prosperous individuals seeking to assist their children who were pursuing Western secular education.[13] Previously, education *abinet* had been confined to religious students.

There are an endless number of stories of individuals whose spectacular success in the business sector, and in religious and governmental institutions was also attributed to the magico-medical assistance they obtained from cleric–healers. Cleric–healers, often referred to as *tanqway*[14] at this time because of their ability to construct magic spells with writing (*tenqwala* means 'to write'), were also said to help prominent individuals, as well as outlaws, to become sharpshooters and impervious to bullets.[15] Cleric–healers, who were renowned for their abilities, developed a regional clientele that required them to travel over considerable distance; for example, to provide magical medicines to the landed gentry, a cleric–healer from Begemder, an *alaqa* ('head' or 'chief of a church'), was constantly travelling to Gojjam and Shewa.[16]

The provision of magico-medical services enabled many cleric–healers to obtain rural agricultural land and political appointments.[17] As a consequence, upward social mobility, not easily attainable during the imperial period, was much more accessible to spiritual and cleric–healers who forged special relations with the aristocratic class, the landed gentry, state officials and local governors;[18] for example, a *tanqway*, who was said to have had a number of high officials and members of the nobility as patrons and beneficiaries, was rewarded in cash and in kind – a house, a car and agricultural land.[19] In addition, the place where the *tanqway* performed his day-to-day services was said to have been provided by one of his clients.[20] The *tanqway* also received protection from his politically and economically powerful clients.[21] When he was accused of taking Holy Communion from a famous church, even though he regularly engaged in impious and idolatrous deeds, security officials took no action against him.[22] The officials' lack of action was due partly to the difficulty of proving such accusations, but also to the fact that almost all the personalities mentioned as the *tanqway's* clients were politically influential and far too powerful for the officials of the Public Security Department to confront. Any conspicuous attempt to do so would have negatively affected their job security and livelihood.[23] It appears that the attitude of the state officials towards the *tanqway* was dictated by expediency rather than principle.

While the upper classes benefited from the powers of cleric–healers, they often portrayed them in a negative light to discourage the majority of the underprivileged public from benefiting from their economically affordable services.[24] Informants stressed that it was out of insatiability, selfishness and jealousy that members of the ruling class deliberately promoted a prejudiced and stereotypical view of church-based healers, while at the same time exploiting and benefiting the most from their multifaceted service.[25] The elites often referred to cleric–healers as ምትሐተኛ *methatagnna*, አስማተኛ *asmatagnna*, ሟርተኛ *muwartagnna*, *aqabe seray*, *tanqway*, *tila wagi*, uncomplimentary adjectives, often colloquial, that were employed to designate church-educated healers as *sorcerers*,[26] *occultists*, *ill-wishers*, and as *murderers* and *possessors of harmful medicines.*

Worse yet, cleric–healers, like their secular counterparts, were also referred to as ሥር ማሽ *ser mashe*, ቅጠል በጣሽ *qital batashe* (literally 'digger', 'cutter', 'collector' or 'picker' of roots and leaves). Derogatory designations for popular and cleric–healers were similar to the pejorative names directed against socially 'segregated' occupational castes: gold and iron smiths, weavers, tanners and potters.[27]

The stigmatisation of cleric–healers was also fostered by practitioners of Western biomedicine, who viewed the clerics as competitors. Many informants claimed that the stigmatisation of cleric–healers and other indigenous health practitioners was particularly severe in areas where Western medicine had been a major source of health care.[28]

Attacks by biomedical practitioners, who often described indigenous medicine as 'primitive', did not go unchallenged. A prominent Ge'ez scholar–healer was quoted as saying: 'There is no such a word as primitive . . . for language and medicine. Even the so-called lower animals: cats, dogs, goats, etc., know more effective medicine against snakes poison and worms than . . . boastful pharmacists and physicians.'[29] Moreover, he claimed that church-based medicine was an ancient therapeutic tradition that deserved to be cherished for the untiring service it had provided for centuries before many scourging diseases had been 'scientifically christened'.[30]

The attacks of Western medical practitioners and the responses of defenders of indigenous forms of healing clearly demonstrated the continued struggle for power and competition for the medical market by proponents of the two medical systems. It should not be forgotten, however, that both secular and cleric–healers had been stigmatised, to some degree, long before the appearance in the early twentieth century of a Western allopathic medical system in the country.

The Change in Attitude of the Imperial Government

In spite of the negative attitudes towards indigenous healers that were fostered by elites and practitioners of Western biomedicine during much of the first half of the twentieth century, at the start of the 1940s the imperial regime began to adopt a much more accommodative stance towards indigenous therapeutics. It is worth noting that the newly restored Ethiopian government did so at a time when most of Africa remained under colonial rule and was dominated by colonial medical systems that largely discounted the value of indigenous healing. Viewing centuries-old medical beliefs and practices as 'pagan quackery', European colonialists banned traditional healing techniques and forced indigenous therapists to go underground. The imperial government's support for indigenous medicine was, in part, a gesture towards preserving the country's cultural heritage, and partly an expression of its support for the anti-colonialist nationalist sentiment that was beginning to spread across the African continent. Cleric–healers played an important role in opposing the Italian occupation. Beyond these nationalist and ideological considerations, however, the state, aware of the dearth of Western-style medical facilities and biomedical healthcare providers in the country, was compelled to tap indigenous therapeutic resources and acknowledge the role of indigenous practitioners in overcoming the country's pressing health problems.

The emperor, whose authority was, as has been shown, augmented by spiritual powers provided by cleric–healers, was a strong advocate of integration. Recognising the importance of indigenous therapeutics for the health of the Ethiopian population, the government issued two proclamations, in 1942 and 1948, which acknowledged the value of indigenous healing methods, while prohibiting any practices that might endanger human life.

Article 8 of Proclamation No. 27 of 1942 reads: 'Nothing contained in this proclamation shall be construed so as to prohibit or prevent the practice of systems of therapeutics according to indigenous methods by persons recognised to be duly trained in such practice provided that nothing in this Article shall be construed to authorize any person to practice any indigenous system of therapeutics which is dangerous to life.'[31]

The new legislation was also designed to control the rapid proliferation of new forms of healing. These included injectionist or 'hybrid' healers, whose diagnostic and therapeutic modalities combined indigenous and Western methods.

Finally, the government also wished to control who could practise indigenous medicine. Thus, the 1948 proclamation established a system of registration or licensing for indigenous healers. At first, individual healers were expected to present themselves to the ministry and have their medication evaluated. This proved difficult because of the Ministry of Health's lack of capacity to understand, let alone evaluate, indigenous practices. Consequently, the minister, Akalework Habtewold, established a committee of physicians to collect information regarding indigenous medical practices and make recommendations about how these practices should be regulated. Specifically, the committee was charged with the task of evaluating each candidate, licensing eligible healers and ending the corrupt practices of certifying unqualified healers.[32] It was also responsible for gathering information and making recommendations on the future growth and development of indigenous medicine.

The committee lost no time in recommending that a research institution for indigenous healers be established along with a legalised healers' association. The association would be fully in charge of evaluating and licensing healers, and responsible for formulating standards and a code of practice, as well as punishment for misconduct and malpractice. The research institute would carry out clinical observations of the effects of therapeutically useful herbs. The committee, while made up exclusively of biomedical physicians, stressed the need to foster dialogue and co-operation between practitioners of allopathic and indigenous medicine.[33] However, the committee found it difficult to discharge its responsibilities, because many indigenous healers employed medicines that could not be easily evaluated. This was particularly true of cleric–healers, whose medical treatments included large numbers of non-herbal medicines, including prayers and written prescriptions. In the long run this would pose a challenge to healers who hoped to gain accreditation under the 1948 legislation.

Worse yet, when Akalework left the Ministry of Public Health in the early 1950s, the work of the licensing committee came to a standstill and the committee was eventually disbanded. The institute for indigenous healers that the committee had proposed failed to materialise.[34] Without the institute, the ministry was unable to implement a system of licensing and evaluation based on knowledge of the ideas and practices of indigenous healers. Instead, the regulation of healers became largely an exercise in prohibiting unlicensed indigenous healers and unlawful users of biomedical products. The licensing procedures were bureaucratic, inconsistent and applied with little understanding of the nature or value of various healing practices. These problems made it difficult for healers to obtain legal recognition.[35]

In order to apply for a licence, a healer had first to obtain a letter of recommendation from the governorate office of the province in which he practised. No healer could present his application to the ministry without first securing a supporting letter from a provincial governor or municipal officer. This was a time-consuming process wherein indigenous healers had to present supporting letters from their respective governors (i.e., district, sub-district or municipalities as in the case of cities) together with written testimonials of individuals[36] verifying the healers' services in their localities for at least the past ten years. Practitioners who had less than ten years' therapeutic experience were not entitled to apply for a work licence. It should be noted that practitioners of Western biomedicine were not required to have worked for such a long period. Several informants suggested that this time requirement was established to limit the number of healers eligible to receive licences.[37]

After meeting these basic stipulations, an indigenous healer had to travel to Addis Ababa to make a formal application to the Ministry of Health.[38] The ministry did not adopt a standard form to be completed by applicants, but it became routine for applicants to present a signed application letter (as in the so-called examination paper) on which his name, age, religion, occupation (other than healing), place of birth, citizenship (including regional or ethnic background), medical experience and current address had to be provided. After evaluating a healer's application and supporting letters, the ministry would determine whether the applicant was eligible to take a so-called examination set by the technical department.

Those who qualified for the examination were required to put down in writing lists of diseases they professed to cure and their corresponding medicaments. One healer, claiming to cure several illnesses, affixed a list of 102 curative herbs to his application letter.[39] Applicants also had to provide information on the aetiology of each and every disease they claimed to be able to treat, the payments they charged for their services (though sometimes omitted), and the manner of administration and 'dosage' of their medicines.[40]

It is interesting to examine the way in which healers' applications were written down and presented. Those who may be referred to as 'overconfident' healers claimed that they wanted to be accredited only after their medicinal herbs were 'scientifically' verified[41] and, if need be, after the curative value of their medicinal herbs had been tested on patients referred to them by biomedical practitioners;[42] for example, an applicant, claiming to possess a dependable therapy for leprosy, elephantiasis and scrofula, expressed his eagerness to demonstrate the value of his herbal remedies to biomedical practitioners. Claims such as these were not uncommon.

While the healers' examinations were in written formats, literacy was not a prerequisite for healers applying for a work licence or to take the examination. Those who could not read or write could enlist the help of a literate individual who would apply on behalf of a non-literate (often secular) healer. Non-literate healers were also allowed to sit for an examination by dictating their responses to a literate person who would complete the examination forms. With the exception of those who refused to provide the ministry with lists of medicines and the illnesses they claimed to cure, almost all the applicants were permitted to sit for examinations and to obtain a work licence.

It was only after meeting the ministry's requirements and standards of practice that an applicant would qualify to obtain a written work permit. An original copy of the permit was issued to the licensed healer, with a carbon copy routinely sent to the provincial governorate offices. The governor's office, in turn, sent copies to lower administrative offices.

The applications produced by healers contained a wealth of information about indigenous healing practices, including the names of botanical remedies. Sadly, the health authorities never analysed them, thereby missing an opportunity for developing fuller knowledge of the potential use of local medications.[43]

Healers not willing to disclose their medicinal prescriptions to the technical department were barred from taking an examination, obtaining a work licence and engaging in a medical practice. Muslim cleric–healers from neighbouring Sudan were among those who were prevented from taking the examination because they refused to disclose their medication. Although these Muslim cleric–healers had qualified to apply for a work licence[44] using supporting letters they acquired from the *Sharia* or Islamic courts, they were adamant about not revealing their medicinal prescriptions to the ministry.[45] This refusal may have reflected the workings of the medical marketplace in Addis Ababa, where most of these expatriate Muslim cleric–healers practised. There was an expanding market for those who could provide alternative therapeutic modalities in Addis Ababa. Within this market the practice, and thus the income, of Muslim cleric–healers depended, in large measure, on the unique qualities of the care they provided. This distinguished them from the large number of Ethiopian cleric–healers and herbalists working in the city and brought them clients. These healers may well have feared that by disclosing the nature of their practices to the Ministry of Health, knowledge of these practices would be disseminated, which would undermine their claim to providing distinct forms of therapy. Though largely unsuccessful, these foreign nationals sought to secure work licences believing that they would be able stay in the market and secure their tenure in the capital. By contrast, local licensed healers understandably opposed the issuing of work permits to foreign medical practitioners, whom they viewed as competing for patients.

The extent to which the technical department of the Ministry of Health could actually evaluate the medication disclosed by applicants in their examinations was questionable. Several domestic healers who provided lists of medicinal plants without mentioning the specific parts or 'dosages' of their herbal prescriptions were not barred from obtaining work licences. In general, the technical department accepted the healers' statements and explanations about their medication and how it worked. Lack of communication and trust between the ministry officials and the healers no doubt discouraged healers from revealing too much about their practices. Many healers presumed that the ministry only wanted to acquire their lists of drug plants and then use them for its own ends.[46]

Nonetheless, a review of their examination papers suggests that the majority of indigenous practitioners attempted to provide a list of their medicines in conjunction with their formula, manner of administration, contraindications and antidotes for adverse reactions. The healers' willingness to reveal the actual medication they employed can be authenticated by comparing the medicines they claimed to use against some common illnesses with medical prescriptions cited in local medical texts. This comparison suggests that healers were not 'secretive' and uncooperative in revealing their medicines to others, as was commonly supposed. Instead, the majority of healers, fearful of losing their work licences (if found guilty of citing incomplete or fake medicines in their examination), seemed to have complied with the request for a truthful and complete list of their therapeutically valuable items. Since there was no single case of an applicant failing his examination on account of presenting an incomplete medicinal list, it is possible that some healers limited the number of drug plants in their lists, perhaps hiding those that they viewed as particularly effective and thus valuable for attracting a clientele.

Interestingly, the ministry accepted examination papers dotted with herbal cures for illnesses allegedly caused by spiritual beings. This was taken by healers to imply that the ministry accepted the mixing of spiritually and naturally caused illness aetiologies and their corresponding cures. As seen from the numerous work licences issued to church-educated healers, the health department did not put in place a mechanism to prohibit licensed church-educated healers from treating illnesses that had non-physical causations. In reality, the ministry's acceptance may well have reflected its less-than-rigorous evaluation of materials presented in the examinations.

Once a healer had passed the examination, he was issued with a licensing letter, which stated: 'In accordance with proclamation number 100 (B) of September 1948 the person referred to above is hereby permitted to provide indigenous treatments not injurious to his patients.' The permission papers made no mention of the specific areas of expertise or modes of therapy the healer was eligible to practise; in other words, there was no effort to limit the licence in relation to the medical knowledge revealed in the examination. The licence therefore provided carte blanche to practise all types of 'indigenous medicine'. This made it very difficult for provincial or district health officials to challenge the claims and activities of healers who possessed a signed and sealed licence from the same ministry or to regulate their practice.

Provincial health authorities in general were sceptical of the whole licensing procedure and its ability to regulate the quality of indigenous healing practices. They noted that no healer would actually admit that his medicines were injurious to health.[47] They also called on the ministry to reconsider its 'unsystematic accreditation' of healers and called for a new evaluation system through which work permits would only be given to a few selected and qualified healers. It seems clear that provincial health officials would have established a more rigorous evaluation process had they been given the responsibility for licensing healers. They resented the fact that they had no say in the evaluation process. Even at the provincial level, it was the provincial governorate offices and not the health offices that provided healers with the letters of recommendation they needed to apply for an examination and work permit. The health authorities, therefore, could not limit the number of applicants.

The aspiration of a handful of indigenous healers went beyond acquiring an accreditation paper; they wished to receive short-term medical training so that they could join the allopathic medical structure and become salaried employees.[48] The ministry did not entertain these requests, saying that it lacked the institutional resources, both technical and human. More fundamentally, the question of partnership was a very challenging issue to the ministry's officials, who perceived indigenous medicine as fluid and unsystematic, and lacking a clearly stated guiding principle or code of ethics to govern healers' actions.[49] In the end, the desire on the part of a few healers to partner with the biomedical practitioners went unrequited.

Many healers were unable to complete the entire licensing procedure, due to financial constraints or because they were discouraged by the complex bureaucratic hurdles they had to negotiate. To complete the registration process, stretching from local administrative offices to the Ministry of Health in Addis Ababa, was in itself more than enough to overwhelm a healer. It is, therefore, not surprising to find that many indigenous healers in rural areas preferred not to comply with the government's regulation and failed to obtain work permits;[50] in fact, the number of indigenous health practitioners working without work licences was believed to be much higher than those who obtained licences.

Unlicensed healers were harassed by local authorities. Along with local injectionists, the unlicensed herbalist–healers were accused of treating patients with unknown or harmful medicines. The police, however, had a difficult time finding evidence to support these charges.[51] Even when they found drugs in the houses of unlicensed healers, they lacked the capacity to determine whether the drugs that were found were harmful. In the end, the police concentrated on identifying whether or not a healer was registered.

Unlicensed healers were also criticised by licensed healers who resented their non-licensed status and wanted to push them out of the medical marketplace. At the same time, licensed healers attempted to use their elevated stature and their accreditation as a marketing tool.

The antagonism of licensed healers towards their unlicensed competitors stemmed from the fact that the general public had little or no information about the registration process, and, hence, failed to distinguish between members of the two classes of healers. Those seeking medical help were concerned with the reputation of the healer for producing a cure for their particular ailment more than with whether the healer was registered. Healers who completed the registration process resented the fact that it gave them little advantage in attracting clients.

The divide between licensed and unlicensed healers, marked by mistrust and suspicion, prevented the formation of a united community of indigenous healers with an organised professional association that would have helped to ensure the collective rights of all healers and solidify their place within the expanding medical marketplace of Ethiopia.

Licensing did not legitimise the work of all indigenous healers. Certain spiritualist–healers, whose therapeutic services were mostly focused on treating non-physical ailments, were viewed by church leaders as potential threats to the spiritual leadership of the Ethiopian Orthodox faith and the security of the state. Officials of the Public Security Department did not officially say that spiritualist–healers were enemies of the state, and the state did not officially prohibit spiritual healers from registering and getting a work licence. The most widespread accusations against spiritual healers were aimed at

Zar shamans, who gathered clients, often in the hundreds, to perform ritual healings commonly referred to as 'moments of revelations or judgments'.[52] Spiritual healers, especially Zar shamans, gained widespread popularity during the imperial era.

These spiritual healers, who were not church-educated, were often referred to as *qallicha*,[53] a term routinely employed to identify individuals known to be possessed and inspired by spiritual beings (though not necessarily noxious ones). The *qallicha* healers claimed to have mystical therapeutic wisdom and were viewed by their clients as being helpful in dealing with a wide range of physical, psychological or psycho-social disorders. Many people brought their personal or social problems to the *qallicha* healers, hoping that they would get an immediate solution or advice on how to deal with their troubles. It was this manifold service that made the *qallicha* attractive to their clients. The spiritual healers were also popular because they dealt with spiritual entities, including the Zar, Buda (evil-eye) and Chele or Atete spirits that did not quite fit into the Ethiopian Orthodox Christian cosmology of disease-causing or misfortune-bearing spirits.[54] The inability of the Orthodox clergy to offer satisfying explanations and treatments for these spirit-caused ailments swayed a growing number of patients to beseech the services of spiritual healers.

The *balazar* spiritual healers, whose expertise went beyond appeasing, cajoling or exorcising spiritual entities, were valued for their advice, guidance and the reassurances they provided to the clientele. They could also diagnose illnesses, including the identification of evil-eyed people and sorcerers held responsible for childlessness and other misfortunes, and provide therapeutic recommendations for a wide variety of physical and mental problems, such as herbal cures, holy water and even biomedical treatment.[55]

The popularity of the *balazar* healers should also be attributed to the instability and disorganisation of the immediate post-occupation period, coupled with the inability of the restored government to provide steadfast security protection, health and other services. This caused the public to seek the services of healers known to be endowed with extraordinary psychic or clairvoyant powers. The situation seems to have been favourable to the coming into prominence of several spiritual healers.

The ability of these spiritual healers to attract large followings threatened the spiritual leadership of the Ethiopian Orthodox Church. Church leaders attempted to suppress these healers by accusing them of practising sorcery and by portraying them as a threat to the state. The clergy claimed that the main goal of these spiritual healers was to attract as many followers as possible to their non-Orthodox Christian, 'idolatrous faith' and ritual practices.

Some of the accusations were communicated through the Office of the Ethiopian Orthodox Church Patriarchate,[56] the highest ecclesiastical office that acknowledged the emperor as a 'guardian of the Orthodox faith'.[57] Sometimes, the Office of the Patriarchate, gathering up complaints from the clergy and other concerned individuals, would write to the Public Security Department – a stabilising force for the imperial regime – requesting it to do something to prevent the laity from being involved in 'idol' worship and detaching themselves from the Ethiopian Orthodox Christian Church.[58]

For example, a very serious charge was brought against an Orthodox *balazar* and a leader of the Zar possession cult, who was said to have undermined the Ethiopian Orthodox Christian faith of the laity of a predominantly Christian community in north Shewa. The *balazar* had held his own 'possession feast' on the day of the Feast of the Epiphany. This limited the participation of the faithful in the Orthodox Feast of the Epiphany.[59] After receiving a report of the incident from a local church, the Office of the Patriarchate sent an appeal to the Public Security Department demanding that the person be punished and his 'irreligious' and non-Orthodox activity be ended.

While the efforts of the clergy to besmirch *balazar* healers as sorcerers appears to have had limited effect on the attitude of the state, reports that these same spiritual leaders were connecting the problems of their followers with the prevailing socio-economic and political conditions in the country drew the state's attention. At possession ceremonies where hundreds of people normally gathered, spiritual healers, inspired by their spirit familiars, are said to have made damaging charges against the state and its policies. This led state officials to tighten their control over these individuals. In a fashion reminiscent of Italian rule, *qallicha* spiritual healers in the immediate post-Italian period came to be viewed by the state as treacherous elements or agents of foreign enemies.

In one interesting case a Ministry of Interior official, gathering reports from provincial authorities, presented a petition to the deputy minister describing diviner monks and the *qallicha* spiritual healers 'as dangerous individuals with a potential to destabilise the state' and claiming that they should be detained and treated just like political prisoners.[60] Stated simply, the *qallicha*, constituting both literate and non-literate soothsayers and diviners, were labelled as dangerous individuals with an enormous potential to upset the status quo of the Haile Selassie regime. Viewing them as a destabilising force, a few provincial administrative officials went so far as to place some spiritual healers under house arrest, others were sent into internal exile.

The treatment of spiritual healers by government officials, however, was inconsistent. State officials reacted strongly to spiritual healers who referred to themselves (often at possession rites) as 'kings', 'lords' or 'governors' of this or that area.[61] Such claims were tantamount to intervening in and/or diminishing the image and accepted authority of the government. However, state authorities refrained from prosecuting spiritual healers for their therapeutic activities. Thus, the head of state security, writing to the Chief of the Police, noted that his department was unable to bring an end to the activities of spiritual healers, whose principal treatment modality of helping the troubled, through the intercessory power of spiritual beings, was no different from the long-established healing method of other healers. During the 1940s and 1950s provincial governors frequently complained that the public security bureau seldom empowered governorate offices to bring the *qallicha* to court.[62] By contrast, some governors and other elites were said to be accomplices of certain spiritual healers, providing them with protection.[63]

Spiritual healers were not the only indigenous healers who were bothered by the authorities; in fact, receiving a licence to practise healing did not free one from the interference of local officials who, as noted above, were often critical of the licensing procedure. The attitude of these officials affected the ability of healers to practise within their jurisdictions.

Before the start of the licensing of indigenous healers in 1948, governors at provincial, district and sub-district level had unlimited power to allow or deny healers permission to work in their respective administrative domains.[64] This absolute autonomy of local rulers, according to Fantahun, was relaxed when work permits were extended to those spiritual healers whose 'prayer' was said to be highly cherished for the wellbeing of the country and the sovereign.[65] Yet local officials continued to have the power to intervene in the lives of indigenous health practitioners and affect their movements. In 1950 a healer claiming to have a 'work licence' from Dessie Municipality with the order of the Crown Prince was not allowed to practise in Addis Ababa because, according to the local authorities, there were more than enough healers in the capital.[66]

A woman with a successful practice in treating several spiritual and physical illnesses claimed that she was accused of intervening in political matters and was forcefully expelled from her home. Unable to get any administrative help from provincial authorities, she was forced to appeal directly to the emperor. Describing the unfair treatment she received from the chief district governor, the woman was anxious to know why he permitted more than 300 *qallicha* to work in his district and why, as she put it, he had 'detained me for a week, shaved my hair, and expelled me from his town without due process of law'.[67] The Public Security Department wrote a letter to the provincial governor demanding evidence that the woman was actually involved in political matters. While the governor failed to prove her political involvement, he insisted that the woman was an impostor who did not have any useful medicine that would in any way help the people of the district.[68] In the end the power of the district governor resulted in the woman being branded as a cheat or a political 'opponent' and not being reinstated to her place of residence.

While the opposition of local authorities could prevent a healer from practising medicine, having the support of a powerful local official could protect a healer from efforts to remove him or her from a local jurisdiction. Thus, when a district governor detained a *qallicha* spiritual healer for allegedly administering unknown herbal drugs and leading the laity to idol worship, the detainee produced written permission from a provincial governorate office and was soon released.[69]

Receiving a permit to work in a particular area did not assure a healer that he or she would not be harassed by the police. A spiritual healer appealing to the Ministry of Interior in the early 1940s wrote that although he had acquired a 'work permit' from the chief district governor, he was deterred from carrying out his duties due to 'constant interference from the police'. He pleaded to the Ministry of Interior to stop this police interference and to provide him with a new work permit. However, the ministry, which was hesitant to become involved in the case, refused to issue the new permit.[70] The ability of local authorities to aid or hinder the work of healers, and the refusal of the Ministry of Interior to interfere in the administration of local cases, left the system for controlling the practice of healers open to corruption and favouritism.

In addition to the challenges healers faced in gaining permission to work in particular areas and avoiding police interference, the penal code provided opportunities for patients to charge healers with malpractice, for which they could be arrested and tried. Article 661 of the penal code entitled 'Fraudulent Exploitation of Public Credulity' threatened practitioners of magic with fines, imprisonment or both. It reads as follows:

> (1) Whosoever, for gain, knowingly deceives another by means such as invoking spirits, magic or sorcery, consulting horoscopes or astrology, by interpretation of dreams, soothsaying, chirography, divining or by any other means of exploiting human credulity, is punishable, upon complaint, with fine, and, in the event of repetition of the offence, with simple imprisonment, where the case does not fall under the provisions regarding petty offenses. (Art. 815).
> (2) Where the deceit is such as to constitute fraudulent misinterpretation, Art. 656 shall apply.[71]

In addition, Article 815 (A) under the heading 'Quackery' reads as follows: 'Whosoever . . . obtains money by taking advantage of the credulity of others by soothsaying in any form whatsoever, by calling upon spirits, is punishable under Article 812.'[72]

These laws, though less valuable to measure the degree of magical beliefs among the Ethiopian public, were aimed primarily at spiritual healers. However, they were particularly difficult to enforce, given the nature of their practices. Charges relating to the realm of the spiritual and cheating the public could not be proven tangibly as most accusers had difficulty finding witnesses (human or material) who could explain or demonstrate objectively how spiritual healers had cheated them or exploited their credulity to the advantage of the defendants. It should also not be forgotten that clients were often hesitant to accuse a spiritual healer for failing to render them proper treatment because the fear of retribution was much higher than the anticipated compensation they would expect from the accused.[73]

By contrast, registered cleric– and non-cleric–healers who administered botanicals were more susceptible to legal charges. Thus, the administration of botanicals allegedly injurious to human health was a *sine quo* for indicting healers under the terms of the penal code described above.[74] Informants noted the injustice of such prosecutions, pointing to the frequent deaths that occurred in hospitals due to malpractice or negligence that were simply overlooked, while a single death at the hands of an indigenous health practitioner was a source of pandemonium and a topic of exaggerated controversy.

Human fatalities were reported to the police; and the police, for their part, laid criminal charges against healers for purportedly causing the death of patients with their medicinal concoctions.[75] Proving the authenticity of such charges was a very complex and lengthy process; specimens of herbal medicines incriminated in the death of patients had to be sent first to the nearby hospitals, then to the ministry's pharmacy department which, in turn, sent them for a chemical analysis to the Central Laboratory; an institution responsible for evaluating the intrinsic nature of specimens.[76]

The dossiers of the Ministry of Interior are filled with cases involving the administration of herbal substances; for instance, a letter written in 1967 noted that herbal specimens, which were allegedly responsible for the deaths of two individuals, were sent to the national laboratory for chemical analysis.[77] The results of the analysis were then submitted to the high court. Interestingly, these dossiers also included discussions about the difficulty of obtaining reliable and conclusive reports from the central laboratory, the lethality, remedial and/or non-poisonous quality of the medicine. Sometimes the manner in which specimens were sent prevented the laboratory from carrying out accurate chemical analyses. These problems made prosecutions difficult to carry out.[78]

Conclusion

While indigenous healers continued to face administrative actions that threatened their ability to practise openly, the Haile Selassie period represented an era of relative openness and freedom for indigenous healers, including church-based healers, when compared to both the earlier Italian era and the post-Haile Selassie period. However, the authority of church-based healing was seriously undermined by the rapid expansion of Western education and literacy, and the growth of printing during the imperial era.

Figure 16: Holder of a written amulet

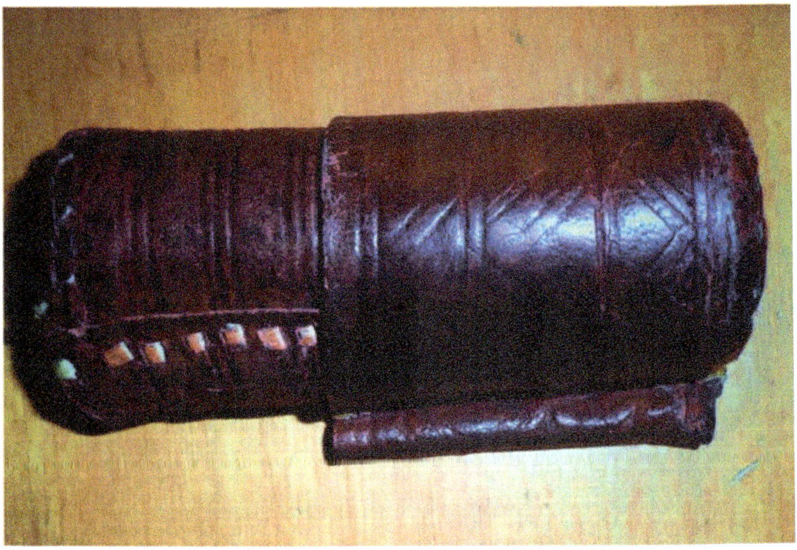

Source: IES Ms. No. 5560

Figure 17: A typical personal amulet to keep the devil and his minions at bay

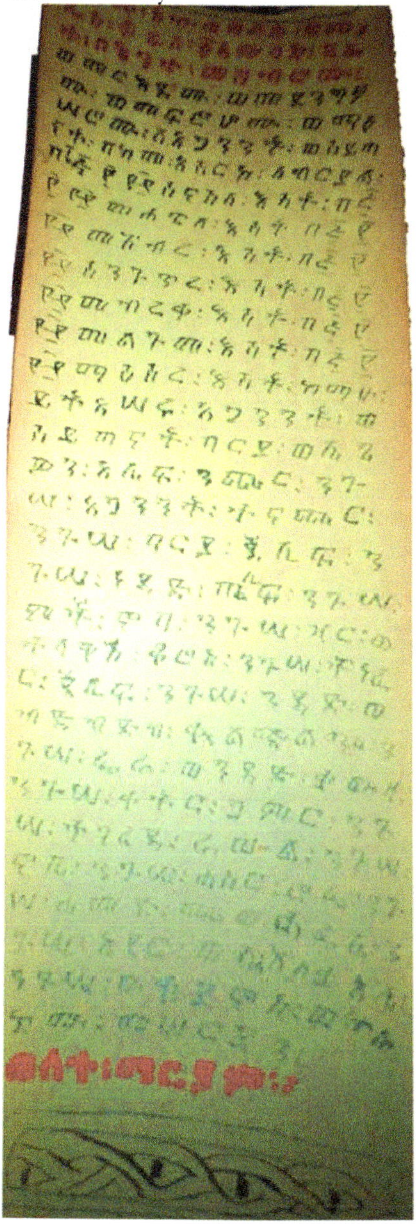

Source: IES Ms. No. 5526

Notes

1 This assertion confirmed what Gebre Hiywot had stated in the early twentieth century. He wrote that there was no one in the whole world like Ethiopian rulers who required the assistance of good and bad spirits. See Gebre Hiywot Baykedagne, *Emperor Menelik and Ethiopia* (Amharic) (Addis Ababa: United Printers, 1993), 5.

2 A corpus of medico-magical texts kept at the Institute of Ethiopian Studies (IES) provides ample evidence on the literate church-based healing methods and the diverse role of cleric–healers. Launched in the early 1960s, the IES library became the principal custodian of religious and magico-medical manuscripts. These manuscripts were acquired from individuals and institutions through purchase or donation; for example, Abba Wolde Tensae (an exorcist–priest working at Woliso, South Shewa, since the 1940s and who died in the early 1990s) donated 185 magic scrolls in the early 1970s; and if one had the chance to go through the list of his patients, the likelihood of getting valuable data on patients' socio-economic background and the spatial distribution of cleric–healers during the imperial period would have been higher. These twentieth-century scrolls had been collected from Abba Wolde Tensae's patients who, seeking to free themselves from the evil influence of magicians and malevolent spirits, were normally required to hand over whatever written magical items they possessed before starting to receive his spiritual treatments. This demonstrated the availability to patients of a couple of therapeutic options – magico-religious treatment from the mainstream clergy and magico-magical healing from cleric or specialist healers.

3 One of the factors attributed to the deposition of Iyassu, who was replaced with Teferi in 1916 as heir apparent to Empress Zewditu, Menelik's daughter, was Teferi's alleged association with the *qallicha* and the magical advice they accorded him. See Zewde Retta, *Tafari Mekonnen: His Long Journey to Power, 1892–1930* (Amharic) (Addis Ababa: Central Printing Press, 1998 E.C), 246.

4 Reidulf Molvaer noted this about this minister who was nicknamed *dabtara* (sorcerer), see 'Medical Anthropology Topics of Relevance', 37; a similar rumour regarding Qorit has been recounted in an Amharic work of fiction entitled *Yabishaftu Qoritoch* (The Limbless at Bishaftu). Tesfaye Gebre Ab, *Yabishaftu Qoritoch* (The Limbless at Bishaftu) (Amharic) (Addis Ababa: Commercial Printing Press, 2001)

5 Tesfaye Gebre Ab, *Yabishaftu Qoritoch*; see also Fantahun Engeda, *Major Political Problems and Struggles During Haile Selassie's Administration as*

Learned from the Biography of the Emperor's Close Associates (Amharic) (Addis Ababa: Berhanena Selam Printing Press, 1997 E.C.), 278.

6 The propinquity of Haile Selassie with people of the church circle, notably hermit monks, was a popular story that exposed his reign to defamatory attacks. Some of the stories circulating about Emperor Haile Selassie predated even his birth. Teferi's detachment from his biological mother immediately after his birth, as well as his secluded upbringing (despite his father's resistance) and his subsequent political prominence, a belief purportedly accountable for creating a rift between Lij Iyassu and Teferi, was said to be a perfect match with the prophesies of several *sheikhs*, including the famous oracle Hussein Jibril of Wore Himano, and hermit monks of Debra Libanos and other monasteries, wrote a long-time public servant and diplomat of the Haile Selassie government, Zewde Retta, *Tafari Mekonnen: His Long Journey to Power*, 1892–1930 (Amharic) (Addis Ababa: Central Printing Press, 1998 E.C.), 18–19, 138–141.

7 A host of prophesies had been circulating around Haile Selassie's downfall. Based on the personal account of an inmate (a *qagnnazmach*) at the Grand Palace in which the military junta had locked up and executed many prominent individuals of the imperial regime, Ahadu Sabure, another long-serving diplomat, wrote that around mid-1973 the aged emperor had sent the *qagnnazmach*, a palace official serving probably as *liqa matane* (a person entrusted to collect, sift and present diviners' prophesies to the attention of the sovereign) to Zeqwala monastery to bring him the prophecy of a hermit diviner about the future of his rule that dominated the country's politics for nearly half a century. Foreseeing the fate of the emperor, the monk accurately told the messenger about the irreversibility of the sovereign's downfall through a military coup in the near future, noted Ahadu. See Ahadu Sabure, *The Downfall of Haile Selassie I and the Rise of the Darg* (Amharic) (Addis Ababa: Neged Printing Press, n.d.), 5–7; Ahadu himself gave credence to the idea that the emperor was always serious in listening attentively to the prophesies of diviners and hermit monks, ibid, 315. For a definition of the term *liqa matane*, see Tilahun Berhane Selassie, *Twentieth Century Ethiopia*, 400.

8 Tilahun Berhane Selassie, *Twentieth Century Ethiopia*, 400–401.

9 See, for example, MS no. 2417 (P).

10 A 115-page magical amulet of the emperor's eldest daughter called *Marbabta Solomon* (literally 'Solomon's Net', a magical prayer to help the bearer get protected from and to bind or defeat demons) can be taken as a single case of cleric–healers' service to members of the court circle. See IES, MS no. 1082.

11 Maxime Rodinson, *Magie, médecine et possession a Gondar* (Paris: Mouton & Co., 1967), 162.

12 Oral informant no. 20. For a brief graphic sociological exposition on litigation, see Teshale Tibebu, *The Making of Modern Ethiopia: 1896–1974*, (Trenton, NJ:, The Red Sea Press, 1995), 134–137.

13 Oral informant no. 18.

14 *Tanqway* would mean literally 'a person who harms others with his evil magical spell' or 'a person who writes with a locally concocted ink using a sharpened tip of reed or feather'. The adjective referring specifically to church-educated literate individuals existed long before the appearance of Western writing tools. It did not include the literate public who developed the art of writing in European-type schools. The verb *tenqwala*, denoting the act of writing, was more appropriate to cleric– than to non-cleric–healers. However, *tenqwala* and *tanqway* in the twentieth century had been interchangeably used to identify both the literate and non-literate practitioners of magic and magical acts in the country. Oral informants nos. 1 and 2,

15 Maxime Rodinson, *Magie, médecine et possession a Gondar*, 164.

16 Maxime Rodinson, *Magie, médecine et possession a Gondar*, 180.

17 Oral informants nos. 11 and 12.

18 The *balazar*, who was put to death by the Italians and identified with a pseudo-military title *fitawrari* (commander of the vanguard), indicated the reciprocal relationship of spiritual healers with the Imperial Court. Ministry of Interior, file no. 29/63, Abebe Desta to the Ministry of Interior, July 1942.

19 Ministry of Interior, file no. 161/1/402, 16 August 1955.

20 It was said to have been located at a place that was very convenient to his clients, including the spouses of important people from the church and court circle, who could visit him without being noticed.

21 An alliance with powerful figures was also a vital tool for cleric–healers to create a web of personal and social relationships. Biniam noted the value of such an alliance in the 1930s, citing a cleric–healer whose relationship with Dajjazmach Abebe Damtew, the son-in-law of Emperor Haile Selassie, assisted him in enhancing his reputation and attracting many clients. See Biniam Weldegebreil, 'Traditional Medicine Practitioners of Addis Ababa: A Historical Account from Imperial Times to the Present', unpublished B.A. Thesis (Addis Ababa University, History 1998), 11.

22 Ministry of Interior, file no. 161/1/402, 16 August 1955; the accused was identified as a person with several magic scrolls around his neck, numbering about 50, according to the accuser's estimate. The accuser also hinted at why this person carried all these scrolls; presumably as a

valuable tool of magical assault and protection, which could be used as material evidence against the accused. The accuser firmly believed that impounding these magic scrolls would be helpful for security officials to reveal the real intentions of the accused who kept on victimising his business competitors and opponents. Added to these allegations, mention was made of the sorcerer who, with the intention of preparing magical remedies to his clients, was said to have roamed around and committed serious crimes against wild animals such as hyenas, monkeys, lizards, snakes, frogs and even birds.

23 Over the past several decades, the idea of magic has been a theme of both folk and 'modern' Ethiopian songs. In the late 1960s or early 1970s, Bahru Qangnaw, in one of his traditional songs, made reference to *madahnitegnna* and *digmtagnna* ('medicine men' and 'magicians'), and the alleged role of herbal and magical medicines in attracting the opposite sex; while Behailu Eshete touched on the supposedly intimate relations of cleric–healers and bar owners (mostly women). Mahmud Ahmed, another popular singer, recommended *mastafaqir* (a love magic) as a potential remedy for the ever-increasing mistrust and enmity among the public.

24 The arbitration of the emperor was said to be required to resolve a dispute between a prominent cleric–healer (a physically handicapped person with consummate magico-medical knowledge and skill) and the one-time governor of Begemdir. During his arbitration, the emperor, recognising the two powerful contestants, was said to have told them that 'they should no more quarrel but to govern the province jointly'. Oral informant no. 30.

25 Oral informants nos. 1, 3 and 45. Informants reasoned that this biased outlook had also affected the stature of church-based medicine and healing. For fear of being stigmatised as ጠንቋይ አምላኪ! (literally 'seer worshipper'), people did not tell about their dealings with cleric–healers. In contrast to this, patients openly visited the *dabtara,* whom Messing referred to as 'uncrowned king of healers in Gondar in the late 1950s'. Simon Messing, 'The Highland Plateau Amhara of Ethiopia', unpublished PhD dissertation (University of Pennsylvania, 1957), 684.

26 Here the word *sorcerer* strictly refers to church-based healers and did not include those who received their magical training outside the church system.

27 An informant's incisive observation illustrated the entrenched attitude of the public towards indigenous health practitioners. He commented: 'It was unfortunate that every hard-working person in the country did not escape from being insulted, despised or mistreated; and the social stigma that sprang out of this unconstructive attitude had an enormous

negative impact on the lives and career of indigenous health practitioners and members of the artisan class.' Oral informant no. 1.

28 Oral informants nos. 41, 42 and 43.

29 Alemayehu Moges, 'Traditional Ethiopian Medicine', 114.

30 Ibid., 121.

31 Its Amharic rendering reads: በዚህ አዋጅ ቅጥል በጥሶ ስር ምሶ ባገሩ እንደተለመደው አኳኋን የሚሰራ ሰው በሥራውም በጣም የታወቀ ከሆነ አይከለከልም:: ይህም ክፍል የሚፈቀደው ማናቸውም ሰው ቅጥል በጥሶ ሥር ምሶ ባገር ልማድ መድኃኒት ለሚያደርግ ነው እንጅ ለሕይወት የሚያስፈራው ሁሉ አይፈቀድለትም። See Imperial Ethiopian Government, *Negarit Gazeta*, A Proclamation Relating to the Registration of Medical Practitioners, no. 27 of October 1942. Proclamation no. 100 of September 1948 reaffirmed the same principle. See Imperial Ethiopian Government, *Negarit Gazeta,* sub-Article 3 (B), 1948. A similar legal provision was made in the 1957 Penal Code; in fact, with the addition of a phrase in Art. 518 (4) which states: 'no such person shall be authorized to practise except amongst the local community to which he belongs'.

32 Asrat Waldayes, 'The Postliberation Period (1941–1973),' in *An Introduction to the Medical History of Ethiopia*, edited by Richard Pankhurst (Trenton, NJ: The Red Sea Press, 1990), 251.

33 Ibid.

34 Ibid.

35 For an interesting account on the licensure of a selected group of African healers, and their ideological and commercial competition with the white biomedical practitioners in Natal in the early twentieth century, see Karen Flint, 'Competition, Race, and Professionalization: African Healers and White Medical Practitioners in Natal, South Africa in the Early Twentieth Century,' The *Society for the Social History of Medicine*, 14(2) (2001): 199–221.

36 Those who provided testimonials also had to put down their names and signatures.

37 Oral informants nos. 1, 2, 24 and 32; legitimacy emanating from a decade-long work experience only helped applicants who had joined the healing profession at least since the late 1930s.

38 Since the 1948 proclamation did not distinguish between various types of indigenous healers and the committee charged with collecting information on indigenous healing practices had not completed its work, the ministry had little reason or ability to apply a preferential system of evaluation which would distinguish one group of healers from another. Hence, the right to apply for a work licence was equally extended to all indigenous health practitioners. This meant not only secular–herbalist healers, but also other groups of healers such as

spiritualist–herbalists and cleric–herbalists, whose therapeutic strategy incorporated herbal remedies, were legible to register. This is abundantly clear from healers' application and 'examination' papers which were suffused with the titles *margeta*, *dabtara*, *alaqa*, *sheikh*, *hajji* (cleric, spiritual healers) and secular ones such as *hakim* (physician) and *ato* (mister). These titles are indicative of healers' religious (Christian or Muslim) and educational backgrounds or qualifications (cleric or non-cleric) as well.

39 Ministry of Health, file no. ቀ-9. A healer had presented an eight-page 'examination' paper containing 31 disease names and their corresponding herbal cures, while another healer presented a three-page 'examination' paper with a list of 10 disease names which he claimed to cure along with the supposed medicinal prescriptions and the payments he demanded from his patients.

40 There are about 422 (probably more) healers' 'application and examination' papers in the ministry's files. Apart from the personal files that can be accessed with difficulty, the Ministry of Health's archives office did not keep a register for recording details of healers according to the types of medical practice they offered. Ibid.

41 Most healers naively believed that differentiating the medicinal value of drug plants, which was perceived as the sole responsibility of the Ministry of Health, was an easy task that could be accomplished in a few days' or weeks' time.

42 Ministry of Health, file no. ቀ-9, 21 February 1948; 6 May 1950.

43 Towards the end of the 1970s the chemistry and economic importance of only two drug plants, *kosso* (*Hygenia abyssinica*), a plant used for the treatment of beef tape worm, and *endod* (*Phytolacca dodecandra*), a molluscide important to control schistosomiasis, had been studied in depth. Until very recently, the situation remained almost unchanged, except for *mettere* (*Glinus lotoids*), another anti-parasitic plant, *gizawa* (*Withania somnifera), gulo zeit* (*Ricinus communis*), *bahr zaf* (*Eucalyptus spp.*) and *dingetegna* (*Taverniera abyssinica*) the efficacy of which have been scientifically ascertained. Despite Ethiopia's classification as a 'world centre of diversity' and the richness of its flora, very little has been known about the 'nearly 500 folk medicinal plants' described by Strelcyn. See Stefan Strelcyn, *Medecine et mlantes D'Ethiopie,* vol. 2; it is also believed that 'there are about 1 000 indigenous species represented in 120 genera of medicinal plants in Ethiopia,' writes Fassil Kebebew. See Fassil Kebebew, 'The Status and Availability of Data of Oral and Written Knowledge on Traditional Health Care in Ethiopia,' *Proceedings of the National Workshop on Conservation and Sustainable Use of Medicinal Plants in Ethiopia*, Addis Ababa, 28 April–May 1998; decades later the

Ministry of Health openly admitted that the abundance of the *kosso* plant did not spare the country from spending more than a million birr yearly to import anti-tape worm medicines. See Ministry of Health, *Proceedings of the First National Conference on Ethiopian Traditional Medicine and Healing* (Amharic), Addis Ababa: 27–29 June 1980. 5.

44 A similar story of prohibition has been reported from South Africa where some Indians working as *inyanga* (herbalist healers), as well as a few whites and coloureds who sought to have legal recognition were denied licences; see Karen Flint, 'Indian–African Encounters: Polyculturalism and African Therapeutics in Natal, South Africa, 1886–1950s', *Journal of South African Studies*, 32(2) (2006): 376.

45 Because of the burgeoning of indigenous health practitioners in the capital, several healers' applications for permission to work in Addis Ababa had been rejected.

46 To collect healers' medicinal prescriptions should not have been an end in itself. The ministry, using its archival documents, could have prepared an indigenous medical text constituting a wide-ranging variety and a nation-wide representation of medicinal prescriptions, including the identification of similar or identical medicaments used in different geographic and socio-cultural settings. It appears, however, that the ministry was not even aware of the existence in its archives of healers' medicinal prescriptions that had been collected since the late 1940s. Moreover, these archival materials may be of importance to identify and measure the degree of complementarities and interpenetrations between secular or popular and cleric–healers' therapeutic strategies. Although stalwartly resisted, in the 1970s the Ministry of Health, once again, attempted to obtain medicinal prescriptions from indigenous healers. In addition to organising healers' associations, the provincial health departments were instructed to collect specimens of medicinal plants from indigenous health practitioners. Ministry of Health, *Proceedings of the First National Conference on Ethiopian Traditional Medicine and Healing* (Amharic), Addis Ababa: 27–29 June 1980, 14.

47 Ministry of Health, file no. ወ-9, Wallo Provincial Health Department to the Ministry of Health, 30 June 1950.

48 Ministry of Health, file no. ቀ-9, 8 April 1952.

49 A similar explanation for the rejection by the Kenyan authorities of traditional medicine has been reported by V. N. Kimani, 'The Unsystematic Alternative: Towards Plural Health Care Among the Kikuyu of Central Kenya,' *Social Science and Medicine*, 15B (1981): 333–340.

50 Many healers working in remote localities may not even have heard about the proclamation.

51 See, for example, Ministry of Health, file no. ቀ-9, Gondar Hospital to Police Station 1, 5 July 1951.

52 It was at the pick of the ritual session that the *qallicha* healers would begin to look into the problem of each attendant and to provide or recommend therapeutic or other appropriate solutions.

53 In the archives of the Ministry of Interior the term *qallicha* was purposefully employed to designate both cleric and non-cleric spiritual healers – Christian and Muslim – as non-religious and idolatrous ones. Next to the *qallicha* the term *tanqway* has been the other widely employed adjective.

54 *Hamar*, Nehassie/Meskerem, 1997 E.C.

55 There is an extensive body of literature on the Zar cult in Ethiopia. Here it may be worth noting the works of a French ethnographer, Michel Leiris, who examined the Zar's psychological and ritualistic aspects, and an American anthropologist, Simon Messing, who analysed its social significance. See Michel Leiris, 'La croyance aux genies "Zar" en Ethiopie du Nord', *Journal de la Psychologie et Pathologique*, 25(1/2) (1938): 107–125; Simon Messing, 'Group Therapy and Social Status in the Zar Cult of Ethiopia', *American Anthropologist*, 60 (1958): 1120–1127.

56 Ministry of Interior, file no. 161/1/402, 16 April 1953.

57 It was with the final consent of the emperor that even lower-level ecclesiastical appointments, such as church administrators, teachers and *margeta* were made practical. See Article 11 of *Negarit Gazeta*, 'Regulations for the Administration of the Church,' 1942.

58 Ministry of Interior, file no. 161/402/7, 16 February 1955.

59 Ministry of Interior, file no. 29/63, 8 February 1944.

60 Ministry of Interior, file no. 2/93, Getahun Berqie to the Vice Minister of Interior, 27 October 1943.

61 Associating the prophesies of spiritualists with anti-Ethiopian foreign elements was a highly exalted issue of the early 1940s; see, for example, Ministry of Interior, file no. 2/93, 29 September 1943.

62 See Ministry of Interior, file no. 2/93, 25 July 1945; file no. 161/1/402 dated 12 July 1951 and 17 October 1953.

63 See, for instance, Ministry of Interior, file no. 161/1/40, 13 August 1951.

64 With the Administrative Regulations Decree no. 1 of 1942 Governors-General were appointed to all provinces by the emperor; and by Decree no. 6 of 1946, the previous *awraja*s were elevated to *teklai ghizat*s, *woreda*s to *awraja*s, *meslene*s to *woreda*s; while the same decree also created *mektel woreda*s that had been abolished in 1960. See Asmelash Beyene, 'Some Notes on the Evolution of Regional Administration in Ethiopia,' *Ethiopian Journal of Development Research*, 9(1) (1987): 37, 40, 41.

65 Fantahun Engeda, *Major Political Problems and Struggles During Haile Selassie's Administration*, 278; conferring healers with a semblance of legitimacy was said to be engineered by Ato Mekonnen Habte Wold (brother of Akale Worq Habte Wold) who, seeing the influx of spiritual healers to the capital, instituted a method of collecting money from spiritual healers to fund the celebrated Agar Fikir Mahbar, an association of performing arts that had originally been founded to counter Fascist propaganda and to cultivate patriotism at the time of the Italian invasion. It appeared that he wrote letters of recommendation to spiritual healers who raised money for the association and to help them obtain work permits from the Ministry of Health; this measure, which was initially introduced to help a limited number of healers to carry on their 'prayers' without any interference from local authorities, encouraged others to do the same. However, in spite of the opposition from the Orthodox clergy to the arguably unilateral action of Mekonnen, trading a work permit for money had been maintained from 1954 to 1958. Ibid., 279–280.

66 Ministry of Interior, file no. ቀ-9, 13 August 1950.

67 Ministry of Interior, file no. 161/1/402, 12 April 1952.

68 Ministry of Interior, file no. 161/1/402, n.d. Though very bold, the woman, using her spiritual familiars, claimed to have a cure for insanity, leprosy, tuberculosis, hepatitis (?), gonorrhea, miscarriage, and a number of therapeutically beneficial magic spells. Another Zar-possessed woman not engaged in healing activity appealed to the Ministry of Interior about the mistreatment she was receiving from the police; and she demanded to be allowed to live in peace with her Zar familiar and without intimidation. Ministry of Interior, file no. 161/1/402, 25 February 1966.

69 Ministry of Interior, file no. 161/1/402, 25 September 1953.

70 Ministry of Interior, file no. 29/63, 11 July 1942.

71 The Imperial Government, Penal Code of 1957. Article 656 penalises healers with 'simple imprisonment or, according to the gravity of the case, with rigorous imprisonment not exceeding five years, and a fine'.

72 Ibid.

73 Since most so-called treatments were not life-threatening, spiritual healers could often escape from criminal responsibility using their claim of providing free medical services to the economically underprivileged class. As seen from Article 518 (3) of the penal code, 'Casual advice, aid or services rendered in cases of urgency or in an emergency or out of kindness or devotion and *free of charge* or the delivery in such conditions of proven and innocuous natural or traditional remedies, do not come under this provision.' Ibid, Article 518 (3) (emphasis added).

74 Ibid, Article 516 which says 'whosoever . . . prepares, gives, sells, distributes or administers to another a potion, powder, philter or any other product or ingredient susceptible of impairing his health, is punishable under Art. 514', that is, 'simple imprisonment not exceeding three months or fine, without prejudice to prohibition of professional practice, if necessary, where the offense is repeated.'

75 Wallo Provincial Health Department, file no. ወ-6, 24 May 1962.

76 This became Pasteur Laboratory in the 1950s, a branch of the Paris-based Pasteur Institute, and with the termination of the agreement with the French, it was renamed the Central Laboratory and Research Institute in the early 1960s. Asrat Waldayes, 'The Postliberation Period (1941–1973),' in *An Introduction to the Medical History of Ethiopia*, edited by Richard Pankhurst, 254.

77 Wallo Provincial Police to the Ministry of Interior, file no. ወ-6, 16 March 1967.

78 The apparent frequency of human causalities resulting from the administration of herbal remedies swayed a provincial health department to remind the Ministry of Health to include in its health education programmes, which was transmitted on national radio, information about the dangers of taking unknown herbal medicines. Wallo Provincial Health Department to the Ministry of Health Pharmacy Department, file no. ወ-6, 2 June 1967. Ullendorff wrote in the 1960s that the national radio had regular broadcasts to educate the public on health and hygiene, and on preventative measures against transmissible diseases. See Edward Ullendorff, *The Ethiopians: An Introduction to Country and People*, 2nd edition (Oxford: Oxford University Press, 1965), 203. In an overwhelmingly agrarian society where the number of people that could own a radio set was dismally small, such an effort had little practical value. It was not uncommon for urban residents to gather around at some selected spots and listen to the various programmes transmitted on the national radio. The same may be true of the relevance of visual health educational materials – leaflets and posters – in 'educating' a predominantly non-literate public.

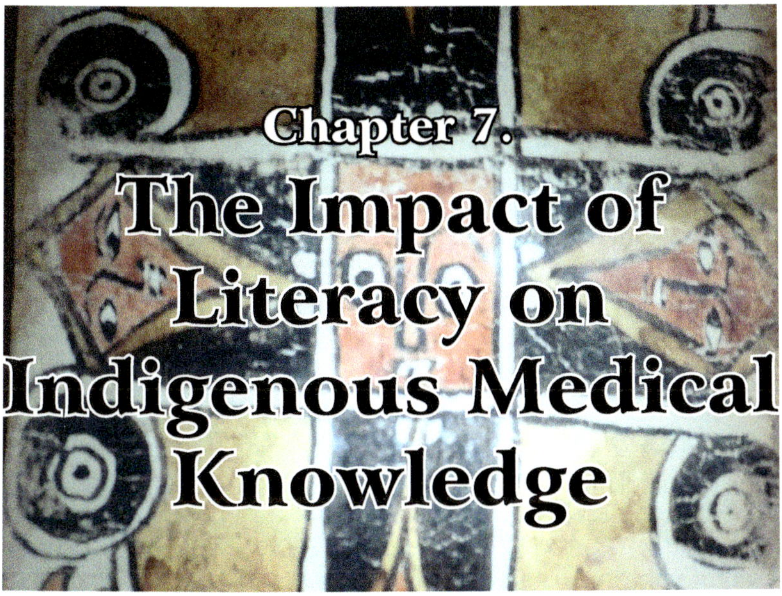

Chapter 7. The Impact of Literacy on Indigenous Medical Knowledge

This chapter examines how the growth of literacy and the proliferation of printing technology affected the time-honoured teaching–learning methods of church-based medicine and healing and, in turn, the status of church-based healers. In the 1920s and 1930s access to esoteric magico-medical texts, knowledge of Ge'ez and the art of writing, were highly restricted and limited primarily to those who had undergone a long and rigorous educational process to become a cleric–healer. Privileged possession of literate skills and written knowledge distinguished church-based healers from other non-Western care providers and legitimised their claims to authority in the medical marketplace. However, the expansion of literacy and printing in the post-Italian era threatened to undermine these claims. This chapter is an attempt to provide insight into the influence of literacy and printing on the diffusion and reputation of church-affiliated medico-magical wisdom.

Expansion of the Art of Writing

Before the Italian invasion, access to the skill of writing had been carefully guarded. Elementary church education provided knowledge of the Ge'ez alphabet, but literacy was restricted. Ge'ez texts were memorised without knowledge of their meaning. It was mostly when students reached the Qene schools that they mastered the ability to write, read and understand the Ge'ez language. It was also at these schools that a few students began to cultivate a close relationship with a learned professor of magico-medical knowledge and, through this relationship, gain access to important medical texts. Students graduating from the Qene Bet could pass on to the Metsehaf Bet where they studied interpretations of the Scriptures, and other religious and secular tracts.

Developing the skill of writing outside these sites of higher learning, either through personal effort or with the help of colleagues and teachers, was viewed as a serious offence. Moreover, providing knowledge of writing illegitimately was viewed by church-based healers as contributing to the dilution of the power of church-affiliated medicine. This was the case because the existence of an increasing number of unqualified 'men of letters' would lead to the injudicious use of magico-medical prayers and prescriptions, and the decline in the importance and power of the written word.

While writing was the avenue through which students gained access to magico-medical knowledge, this access was dependent on developing a close relationship with an existing church healer who possessed medical texts. Cultivating this relationship was an arduous exercise, which could take years to achieve.

Thus, the privileged power of church-based healing was preserved through limiting access to literacy, on the one hand, and magico-medical texts, on the other. In the wake of the Italian invasion, both of these gate-keeping mechanisms were partially breached, first, through the expansion of Western-based education, which opened up access to literacy to a much larger population, and, second, through the development of new printing technology, which made certain religious-medical texts more widely available.

The monopoly of church-trained scholars over the written word and thus over magico-medical knowledge was partly undermined by cleric–healers themselves. Cleric–healers felt obliged to divulge to popular/secular healers a limited number of the herbal prescriptions drawn from magico-medical texts, in order to acquire direct, as opposed to written, knowledge of local plants and herbs. Cleric–healers asserted that they spent considerable time studying the 'hypothetical' value of numerous herbal prescriptions from medical texts, many of which were not even tested or proved efficacious. They believed that unless they obtained the requisite knowledge of how to differentiate botanical remedies and their proven therapeutic value, knowing disease names and prescriptions from medical texts by themselves was not enough to become an accomplished cleric–healer. As one healer noted: 'Once we learnt the names of medicinal herbs from Ge'ez magico-medical texts, it was not difficult for us to differentiate their true identity and their curative importance from the lay people.'[1] Yet this exchange of Ge'ez prescriptions for botanical knowledge detached medical prescriptions from magical prayers and diminished the putative importance of the magical use of the written word (a principal source of church-based healing). At the same time, it led to the dissemination of magico-medical knowledge to non-cleric–healers. These exchanges were much less threatening to their control of magico medical knowledge than were advances in education and printing, beginning with the Italians. These developments greatly accelerated the expansion of literacy and popular access to magico-medical knowledge.

The post-Italian period saw the expansion of Western education and the appearance of a growing number of literate individuals in the country. This expansion of literacy did not immediately lead to an increase in the number of people who had access to magico-religious texts and thus to the knowledge of church-based healers. This is because Amharic was the only local language offered in Western schools. Thus Western education did not increase access to Ge'ez, which was essential to the acquisition of magico-medical knowledge. However, many of those who had acquired knowledge of Ge'ez, as well as some knowledge of magico-medical texts, through religious training, went on to enter Western schools. Religious students, in fact, did well in Western schools. This pattern of dual education made possible the wider dissemination of magico-religious knowledge. By being literate in both Amharic and Ge'ez, these students were able to translate Ge'ez medical texts into Amharic and make them accessible to a population that was becoming increasingly literate in Amharic.

These bilingual individuals who had acquired a limited amount of magico-medical knowledge during their stay in religious institutions were instrumental in the wider dissemination of church-based medical knowledge in Amhara society. Many of these literate individuals, using written source materials independently and without the help of church-educated literati, portrayed themselves as church-trained healers. Others who became teachers in Western-style elementary schools passed their limited magico-religious knowledge on to their students or colleagues.

From the perspective of established church-based healers, the appropriation of medical or magical knowledge through unconventional methods led to 'the transmission of below-standard medical knowledge'. Those who acquired medical knowledge outside formal institutions, which had trained an elite group of church-based healers for generations, obtained partial knowledge of medical practice that involved, primarily, knowledge of herbal medication. However, herbal medication and prescriptions alone were insufficient. For this knowledge would not allow them accurately to diagnose the spiritual or psycho-social side of their patient's problems. To do this, it was essential for a cleric–healer to have a basic knowledge of manipulating alphabets, numbers and divinatory texts. Divination (especially an aspect of 'onomancy' or 'divination through calculation based on names')[2] enabled a healer to look into a whole range of aetiological categories, to figure out the horoscope of his client, spot the responsible ailing agent(s) and to provide appropriate cures. One of the most serious drawbacks of non-church-affiliated healers has been their lack of knowledge of the non-physical aspect of illnesses, and the interconnectedness of the physical and spiritual aspects of most illness episodes; a perplexing situation that might be dealt with concurrently or one after the other.[3]

Cleric–healers were particularly sceptical of healers who had not been formerly trained in the reading and writing of Ge'ez texts but had, instead, acquired their knowledge from texts translated into Amharic. These so-called book openers possessed dubious theoretical and technical mastery of astrological or divinatory treatises and were, therefore, unable to offer proper solutions to their clients.

Those who did not have intensive training in Ge'ez grammar, including its complete sets of alphabets and the system of numerals, 'had little more than jargon-ridden knowledge . . . [and] could not even understand the meaning and purpose of every single word inscribed in a divinatory text'.[4]

Instruction in the writing and manipulation of the Ge'ez alphabet and numerals was what provided medical students with the ability and confidence to consult and exploit divinatory and magico-medical texts.[5] It was only after a long period of intensive study and the assistance of experienced cleric–teachers that a select few literate students had been able to develop these skills and become cleric diviners.

For cleric–healers, the expansion of literacy also aggravated the problem of misusing alphabets. Those who dabbled in Ge'ez texts and sought to manipulate numbers and the alphabet without proper training were bound to make mistakes and, in doing so, discredit proper church-based astrological–medical practices, as well as potentially cause harm to their clients. This problem was exacerbated by a proposal, first put forward in the 1920s, but then pushed by Western-trained scholars at mid-century, that the Ge'ez alphabet should be simplified, so that it could be made more accessible. The proposal created a rift between those who had profound church education and those with little or no church education. To most church scholars and cleric–healers alike, the idea of trimming down the alphabet in the name of orthographic or linguistic standardisation was equated with a 'genocidal act'[6] of irresponsible individuals.[7] The few characters that sounded the same were believed to have distinct meanings, numerical representations and purposes.[8] 'As in their shapes, characters have distinct sounds, secrets and names, and they should be differentiated let alone while being inscribed but also while being read,' wrote a prominent church scholar.[9] To be able to utilise each and every alphabet in a proper way, an indispensable skill to draw on divinatory texts and to work as a cleric–diviner, a student must receive rigorous instruction from an educated mentor. Otherwise, he would be liable to commit serious mistakes. Incorrect use of the alphabet in identifying names of human beings, specific illnesses or disease-causing spiritual entities could lead the unqualified to make a faulty diagnosis and application of medico-magical prescriptions. This would, in turn, produce unwanted or deleterious effects.[10]

In summary, from the perspective of cleric–healers, the spread of literacy expanded access to church-based medicine at the same time that it threatened to undermine its integrity. Expanded literacy allowed book openers to use divinatory texts improperly for diagnostic or therapeutic purposes, while efforts to simplify the alphabet made the manipulation of letters and numbers without proper training a dangerous proposition. All these changes threatened the medical dominance of cleric–healers and undermined the integrity of church-based astrological wisdom.

Modern Printing vis-à-vis Indigenous Technology

While the expansion of literacy provided an increasing number of people with the tools for practicing magico-medicine, the flowering of Western printing technology, beginning in the 1920s, made available some religious and medico-religious texts that had previously only been available to a limited number of church scholars.

Before the 1920s, medico-religious texts had been produced by hand by a small number of advanced church students who were able to acquire writing skills. The few copies that were produced in this manner were closely guarded by legitimate cleric–healers. This situation began to change with the work of Tesfa Gebre Selassie who launched a private printing firm in the 1920s to publish purely religious, magico-religious and historical texts.[11] Tesfa Gebre Selassie was church-educated and started his career by selling hand-written religious texts around 1915/16. Tesfa was best known for his popular banner: 'Let knowledge expand, and ignorance be eliminated'.[12] Tesfa's printing press, named after him, was fully engaged in publishing and making available printed materials ranging from pocket-size Ethiopian alphabets and magico-religious texts to voluminous religious and historical books. Dispossessed of his printing machines during Fascist Italy's occupation in the mid-1930s, Tesfa discontinued printing until 1953 when he acquired a new printing machine and returned to publishing. He collected his materials for printing through wearisome copying, borrowing or purchasing; and for that purpose he travelled to numerous churches and monasteries.[13] One of Tesfa's goals was to provide the poor with prayer texts at an affordable price.

Many of the materials that Tesfa Gebre Selassie published, beginning in the early 1950s, were magico-religious texts. Among them 'Lesane Sab' (Prayer against Backbiters or Slanderers), *Lefafe Tsedeq*[14] (*Bandlet of Righteousness* or *Ethiopian Book of the Dead*), 'Mashafa Bartos' (Prayer of St Mary at Bartos), *Mashafa Tuladan* (*Book of Tuladan*), 'Asmata Malakot' (Secret Names of the Divinity), 'Temherte Hebuate'[15] (Lessons on Mystery), 'Tselote Aqabe Rees' (A Prayer to Protect Oneself), 'Magrarie Tser[16] wa Girma Moges' (A Prayer to Defeat One's Foe and Being Respected), 'Selote Baenta Aynatila wa Shotalay wa Mastafaqir' (A Prayer Against the 'Shadow of the Eye' and Miscarriage, as well as to Be Loved), 'Girma Moges wa Mastahafir' (A Prayer to Be Respected or for Charisma and Being Feared), 'Malka Giyorgis, Mikael, Gabriel, Ruphael, Ragueal' (Prayers in the Image of Saints George, Michael, Gabriel, Raphael and Reguel), 'Dersana za Arbaatu Liqane Malaeket' (Homilies of the Four Archangels: Michael, Gabriel, Raphael and Reguel) and 'Dersana za Sabatu Liqane Malaeket (Homilies of the Seven Archangels: Michael, Gabriel, Raphael, Reguel, Phanuel, Satueal and Afnean) may be cited as outstanding examples. Many of these prayer books consisted of the secret names (or *asmat*)[17] of saints and angels with or without talismanic drawings, and were specifically produced to help the bearer triumph over and protect him or her from myriads of illnesses and misfortunes.[18]

Tesfa often published prayers that were extracted from longer religious and magico-religious manuscripts, which he had copied intact. These shorter texts were printed in large numbers and were sold cheaply. This practice made the prayers available to a wider readership and, no doubt, increased his profits. Critics, however, complained that Tesfa's method of producing shorter prayers from larger ones was an unacceptable practice. The unavoidable omissions and reductions occurring during the publishing process made the 'transmission of magico-medical knowledge deficient'.[19]

The wide distribution of magico-religious texts through Tesfa's publishing activities was a source of apprehension to well-educated cleric–healers. While some healers acknowledged that the wider availability of texts made possible by printing could benefit properly trained healers who would otherwise only have had access to a few magico-medical texts, most cleric–healers worried about printed magico-medical texts coming into the possession of individuals with little or no Ge'ez education and training. They believed that learning magico-medical subjects through self-instructive methods and without the assistance of a learned healer was no more than a self-deceptive act, which could lead to self-destruction. Students who possessed copied medico-magical treatises had to obtain guidance and instructional support from experienced cleric–healers.[20]

Cleric–healers also opposed the publication and diffusion of medical texts, including glossaries of the Ethiopian flora and medicinal plants that began to appear in a printed form in the 1960s,[21] because they saw them as undermining the proper education of young healers. Youthful cleric–healers were attracted to the published medical texts for they assisted them in learning about drug plants single-handedly. As one cleric opined: 'It is still advantageous to have a copy of these texts principally for those who need to learn more about the indigenous herbal therapy.'[22] Not surprisingly, this same ease of access to published medical texts was viewed by more senior healers as a barrier to the education of those trying to learn the practice of church-based healing. They argued that reliance on printed materials prevented healers from making use of unpublished medical texts and from cross-checking the validity of medicinal prescriptions by comparing sources. Reliance on published texts also deterred students from seeking out 'proven' or 'tasted' drug plants from other learned cleric–healers. Finally, they argued, too much faith in a limited body of phytotherapeutic knowledge derived from few printed texts undermined the professional role and reputation of healers working in the medical field.[23]

Experienced cleric–healers quite often warned their students about the danger of gullible reliance on printed medical texts that would make their medical knowledge unfulfilling and untrustworthy at the same time. Even students who possessed inherited medical texts were strongly advised to work with learned healers and to develop their medical knowledge in congruence with the time-honoured instructional methods; for instance, drug plants with multiple appellations often put medical students at risk of committing serious mistakes, argued cleric–healers; and in order to circumvent this problem, medical students should get intensive theoretical and practical instruction on how to differentiate the true identity of drug plants in Ge'ez, as well as in additional local languages, and commit it to memory. All of these arguments, of course, were self-serving in that they came from senior cleric–healers whose status stemmed from their claim to being the only true repositories of magico-medicinal knowledge.

Concerns about the threat that printed medical texts represented to the status of formally trained church-affiliated healers can be seen in contemporary attitudes and reactions towards the *Awda Nagast*, a text originally published in the late 1940s and reprinted half-a-dozen times up until the early 1970s. It appears that the main data in the *Awda Nagast* came from a series of articles (apparently translations of Ge'ez manuscripts) published in an Amharic newspaper called *Voice of Eritrea* by a writer named Temesgen Gebre. It may be argued that the publication of the *Awda Nagast* was a breakthrough in the history of church-based medicine and healing, because it made the mystified wisdom of church-based diviner–healers widely available for the first time. The event was followed by the publication of several printed herbal medical texts over the next three or four decades. The *Awda Nagast* may be seen as a response to the growing demand for published medico-magical or divinatory texts among the limited number of church-educated literati, students of the healing arts and a section of the Ethiopian public.

Yet the publication of *Awda Nagast* was problematic in several ways. First, the popular text was not always published in its entirety. An abridged version was printed with a 1953 E.C. (1960/61) publication date and no mention was made of the original editor and publisher.[24] This version may have been intended to provide would-be astrologers with a user-friendly text that included only the most important parts of the original text. No one knows for certain why the undisclosed publisher did this, and why the intellectual and moral rights of the original editor/publisher were not protected by law.[25] Yet the publication of this version demonstrated that once an important medical text was published, it was subject to a range of modifications that could radically distort its original meaning and purpose. Yet even in its complete form, the publication of the *Awda Nagast* generated considerable concerns for mainstream Orthodox clergy and cleric–healers.

According to Melaka Berhan[26] Admassu Jembere, a distinguished *qene* scholar, the publication of the *Awda Nagast* was an outright heretical act by the editor, Zamanfas Qedus, whom he described as an 'insatiable person'.[27] The editor of the *Awda Nagast*, a protestant, had written a previous book in which he had attacked vociferously the creeds, rituals, apocryphal and other religious texts of the Orthodox Church. His motivations for publishing the *Awda Nagast* were clearly suspect, and Jembere accused him of attempting to humiliate and portray the Orthodox Church as a hub of sacrilegious literature. Jembere had also written a rejoinder to the editor's first book. Jembere accused the editor of being a sorcerer who disguised his true intentions in the name of proving the futility of divination and sorcery while he was avidly interested in propagating the art of divination and sorcery among the public.[28]

In point of fact, the editor of the *Awda Nagast* stressed that it was necessary to publish the text at the time when divinatory treatises were in short supply and accessible only to a few literate individuals. He published the text believing that it would help the literate people get access to this highly guarded but hollow 'wisdom'. The editor's purpose was, in effect, to disseminate the text, not to encourage the spread of church-based medical knowledge but to discredit it. According to Zamanfas Qedus, astrology was an evil wisdom initiated and propagated by the descendants of Cain, and whose wicked teaching included the art of digging roots and preparing herbal medicines along with the skill of manufacturing destructive tools such as swords, lances, spears, bayonets, knives, bows and arrows.[29] *Awda Nagast* 'has been published to unveil the evils of the [religious] student,' asserted the editor, and to help the public obtain its own copy and free itself from the grip of so-called knowledgeable persons. Irrespective of their ecclesiastical positions, he criticised the learned clergy bearing the title *Alaqa*, *Mamhir*, *Kagnegeta*, *Gerageta* or *Dabtara* as incompetents who failed to offer the least desirable solution to the problems that beset the contemporary world, while, as he put it, prominent academics openly admitted their weaknesses and stressed the importance of additional investigations to learn more about the secrets of nature.

Qedus, quoting from Enoch (2: 1–25) and Genesis (4: 22), condemned the Orthodox scholars and cleric–healers for not teaching the truth to the faithful and keeping this worldly wisdom or 'wisdom of death' in secret. To support his argument, Qedus quoted Kidane Wold as saying: የዛሬ ዘመን ባህታዊ ላዩ ሰንሰለት በውስጡ ግን ዐውደ ነገስት። (literally. 'The hermit monk of our time is tied with chains overtly while he carries *Awda Nagast* covertly').[30] Qedus, emphasising the ideology of endless universal struggle between God and Satan that stood for the good and evil or the wisdom of death and life respectively, wrote that many church people, being vulnerable to the temptations of Satan, had become busy pursuing the wisdom of death.[31] He offended the clergy by telling the public to discriminate between so-called pious or religious persons and those who kept on doing this sinful deed unashamedly. For this, he applied the dictum: 'If you do not know that a person is leprous, you may eat together with him.' Such an insult that openly tarnished the hard-won medico-magical wisdom of cleric–healers ignited endless debate and controversy.

The degree of anger created by the publication of the *Awda Nagast* is apparent in the fact that criticisms against the book continued unabated decades after its first appearance in a printed form in the 1940s.[32] One of the strongest critics was Alemayehu Moges, a theologian and cleric–healer. More than using his text as *lurci causa*, Moges criticised the editor as a person interested in 'destroy[ing] anything Ethiopian and Orthodox both good and evil [and] in propagating the new coming [sic] missionary beliefs.'[33] Moges believed that the editor made his defamatory propaganda 'under the cover of philosophical, theological and cultural reformation'.[34] Though his arguments had the flavour of defending the fundamental creeds and teachings of the Orthodox Church, Moges's paradigm clearly reflected the degree of conservatism and mysticism surrounding the medico-magical knowledge of cleric–healers. While cleric–healers criticised the publication of the *Awda Nagast* as an attack on the beliefs and practices of the Orthodox Church, the appearance of divinatory/magico-medical literature in printed form outraged cleric–healers because it impinged on their monopoly over the healing arts. Informants conceded that dissemination of medico-magical ideas through Western technology posed a serious threat to the nearly exclusive control over the written word of cleric–healers.[35]

Many cleric–healers rejected the publication and dissemination of medico-magical and divinatory texts on the grounds that the availability of such texts to the public contravened the time-honoured 'standards and procedures' with regard to safeguarding and transmitting church-affiliated medical knowledge and practice. They cautioned that accessing these texts would encourage the untrained to apply medico-magical information haphazardly, which could inflict serious health hazards upon themselves and others. They also stressed that putting local medico-magical texts in print would not in any way benefit the country. However, it could provide an opportunity for those who sought to exploit the country's indigenous medical heritages without proper compensation.[36] It is worth noting that those who made these remarks did not know that several scholarly investigations, translations and publications in scholarly journals of Ethiopian magico-medical prayers and prescriptions had been carried out before and after the Italian invasion.[37]

The criticisms of cleric–healers may have had some restraining effect on those who wished to publish medico-magical texts in subsequent decades, for few published medical texts appeared in the post-*Awda Nagast* era, even though the technology of publishing became cheaper and more widely available. Nonetheless, a few texts did appear.

Haddis Gebre Meskel, an apparently church-educated Ethiopian, edited a small medical manuscript in Amharic in 1988.[38] The manuscript that Meskel edited was looted from Maqdala in 1868 and kept in the British Museum (as Orient 829) for more than a century. A similar manuscript, investigated by Stefan Strelcyn, was published in the *Journal of Ethiopian Studies* in the mid-1960s.[39] Meskel noted that 'this text which appears to have been written down at the start of the nineteenth century must be a translated copy of a text written before several years [or centuries?]'.[40] He also underscored the importance of conducting research and bringing to light the secrets of ancient Ethiopian manuscripts. Similar to Strelcyn's article written in a foreign language, and meant for researchers and academicians, Meskel's medical text, which was published in a private press in Britain and with a small print run, has been little known outside of the IES library.

Ahadu Ayehu was another church-educated scholar–healer who compiled a 300-page Ge'ez–Amharic medico-magical text. The special working relationship he had with the Ethiopian Studies Institute enabled him to work for years on an anthology of the institutes' medico-magical manuscripts. In preparing his magico-medical text, Ayehu adopted the time-honoured, church-based methods. As seen from his introductory notes, he stressed the significance of spawning a text that contained both herbal and magical prayers and prescriptions. The author, a protagonist of the inseparability of magic prayers and medical prescriptions, argued that it was through the permutation of these two healing methods that cleric–healers in the past achieved considerable success with many physical, mental and social problems.[41] Unfortunately, Ayehu's unpublished type-written manuscript was destined to the IES library and to be accessed by only a very few researchers. The text might have been published and disseminated had the compiler not died a few years later.

Another less well-known, unpublished herbal pharmacopoeia that predated Ayehu's text was prepared by Leul Wolde Ruphael. This hand-written herbal medical text of the early 1980s has been the only single local medical text kept at the National Library in Addis Ababa. The writer avowed that he prepared this text in which he noted down illnesses, physical and non-physical, and their corresponding herbal cures after touring around Gondar, and consulting numerous cleric–healers and medical manuscripts.[42] Even if he had copied medico-magical prayers and prescriptions from several cleric–healers, he kept them for himself. This person claiming to have had church-based medical education appeared to be interested in including medico-magical healing methods in his text, but the political situation did not allow him to do that.

In addition to the expansion of literacy and the development of new printing technology, the integrity of church-based healing and the legitimacy of cleric–healers were challenged by the appearance of factory-produced paper and ink. Cleric–healers maintained that the introduction of factory-produced paper and ink led some healers to ignore the value of traditionally prepared inks. This, in turn, had led to a decline in indigenous writing methods and in the efficacy of written *abinet.* Cleric–healers believed that providing patients with magical prayers on a piece of parchment vellum written by a traditionally prepared ink known generically as እፍራን ቀለም *efran qalam* (the seven principal colours),[43] together with other ingredients, was an effective strategy for coping with many ailments and complaints. With the arrival of factory-produced paper and ink, however, many so-called cleric–healers, being insensitive to the value of *efran qalam* and to the nature, character and meaning of words, simply inscribed magical prayers using non-indigenous writing items.

Despite these problems, the proliferation of factory-produced paper and ink in the twentieth century did not render the indigenous technology entirely obsolete. For much of the post-Italian period, many cleric–healers taught students who were willing to take the trouble of going through the time-honoured training processes.

Conclusion

For much of its history, the control of church-based medical knowledge by cleric–healers was ensured by their privileged access to the skills of reading and writing Ge‘ez, and their special ability to manipulate letters and numbers. Literacy, and particularly the skill of writing, was highly restricted in Amhara society, and acquiring both took years of training. Cleric–healers also maintained their control of medical knowledge through the guarded possession of magico-medical texts. The spread of literacy, beginning with the Italian occupation and accelerating during the Imperial era, together with the development of printing, leading to the proliferation of translated medical texts, threatened both the integrity of church-based medicine and its control by cleric–healers. As a result, while indigenous medical knowledge was recognised by the imperial government, the place of church-based healing was not improved. This combination of official recognition, combined with a decline in the integrity and dominance of church-based healing, continued following the revolution which toppled the Haile Selassie regime in 1974 and brought to power a Marxist military regime that sought to recognise indigenous healing while stripping off its religious roots.

Figure 18: A talismanic art on a personal amulet

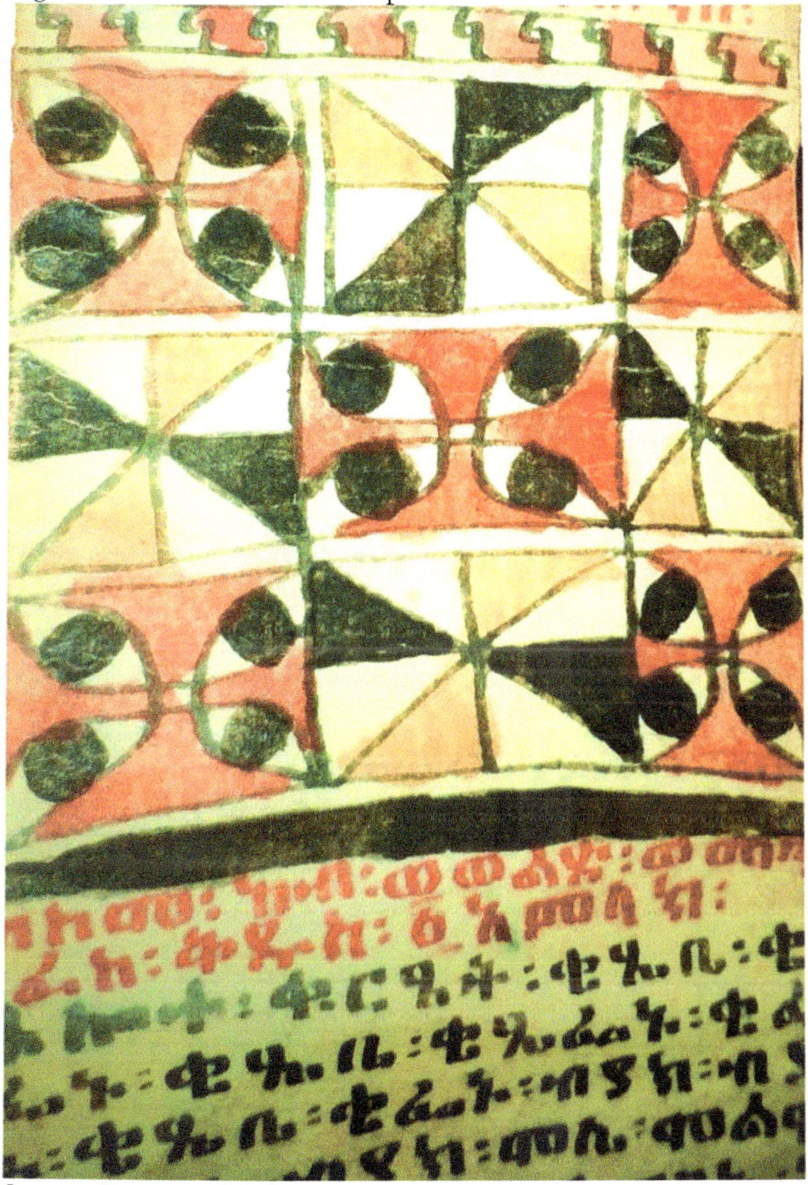

Source: Courtesy of IES

Notes

1 Oral informant no. 2.

2 Richard Kieckhefer, *Magic in the Middle Ages* (Cambridge, Cambridge University Press, 1989), p. 89.

3 Oral informants nos. 2, 8, 20, 30 and 35.

4 Oral informant no. 37; for an interesting discussion on the nature, character and the need for conservation of the Ethiopian alphabets, see Ermias Kebede (Nebura Ed), *Ethiopia: For the World to Judge* (Amharic) (Addis Ababa: Berhanena Selam Printing Press, 1993 E.C.), pp. 412-413.

5 Confirming this assertion Weissleder in his dissertation on the Manz Amhara comments, 'books that give control over demons and spirits are ... [also] accessible to ... [l]earned laymen who have progressed beyond a certain point in their traditional church schooling [and they] can acquire the capability, if they can get hold of the books and have the courage, to get directly involved with the perilous creatures of darkness.' Wolfgang Weissleder, 'The Political Ecology of Amhara Domination', unpublished PhD. dissertation (University of Chicago, 1965). p. 78.

6 Leykun Berhanu, *Tsetset* (Remorse) (Amharic) (Addis Ababa: Neged Printing Press, 1999 E.C.), p. 23.

7 Kidane Wold Kifle, *Book of Grammar and the New Ge'ez Etymological Dictionary* (Amharic) (Addis Ababa: Artistic Printing Press, 1948 E.C.); Desta Tekla Wold, *New Amharic Dictionary* (Amharic) (Addis Ababa: Artistic Printing Press, 1962 E.C.); Ermias Kebede, *Ethiopia: For the World to Judge* (Amharic), pp. 401–419; for a very brief technical explanation on the misuse of alphabets, see an Orthodox bi-monthly publication called *Hamar*, May/June, 2003. Those who favoured the reduction scheme have been referred to in the literature as 'surrogates of historic enemies of Ethiopia' whose real motive was far more destructive than the mere destruction of the Ethiopian alphabets.

8 In the early 1930s Griaule demonstrated the role of the alphabets in Ethiopian divination; see Marcel Griaule, 'Notes sur l'arithmomancie ethiopienne,' *Journal de la Societe des Africanistes* IV (1934).

9 የድምፅ ልዩነት አላቸውና ሚስጥራቸውና ስማቸውም እንደመልካቸው እየቅል ነውና ስንኳን በጥፈት በትምህርትም ባገሳሰስም ሊለዩ ይገባል። Kidane Wold Kifle, *Book of Grammar*, p. 7. The same may be true of repetitive words (mono or polysyllabic), symbols and phrases that have frequently been used in magical prayers and referred to as unintelligible. However, Grebaut noted that በመጽሐፍ ፀሎት በከታብ ቢሆን የሚገኘው ቃል የሚታወቅ ነው፡፡ የማይታወቅ ቃል የለም ከሊቃውንቶች የመጣ ነው የተማረ ያውቀዋል ያልተማረ አያውቀውም እንጅ። (literally 'The so-called unintelligible words in prayer books or written amulets as handed down from previous scholars have

been well known to the learned and unknown to the uneducated'). See, Sylvain Grebaut, *Recueil de texts magique Ethiopiens*, p. 15. The pervasiveness of this problem must have persuaded Wallis Budge to comment boldly that '[s]ome of the best written and oldest amulets of Ethiopia . . . are sheer nonsense.' See Wallis Budge, *Amulets and Superstitions* (London, Humphrey Hilford, 1930), p. 186.

10 Oral informant no. 1.

11 The famous printing press Berhanena Selam (Light and Peace) was founded by Ras Teferi, the future Haile Selassie I, in 1920. It is also worth noting the establishment around the early 1940s of Tensae Zagubae, a new printing press owned by the Orthodox Church., which began to publish and distribute several Ge'ez and Amharic religious texts.

12 Wossen Debebe, *Tesfa Gebre Selassie of Bulga* (Amharic) (Addis Ababa: Tesfa Gebre Selassie Printing Press, 2004 EC), p. 52.

13 For a general treatment of the subject, see Seyfu Admassu, 'Tesfa Gebre Selassie and His Printing Press' (Amharic), unpublished B.A. Thesis, (Addis Ababa University, ILS, 1987). Tesfa's claim of publishing prayer texts was targeted at providing the laity with መንፈሳዊ ምግብ (spiritual food) and helping the poor buy these prayers at affordable prices. As seen from the prices of published prayers, the idea of helping the poor was, in fact, one of the objectives of Tesfa.

14 Responding to Zamanfas Qedus Abraha's criticism of the apocryphal texts of the Orthodox Church, Admassu Jemberre argued that the use of *Lefafe* had never been officially endorsed by the church and to make use of this magico-religious prayer as a personal amulet had been the choice of individuals. Admassu Jembere, *Kokeha Haimanot* (Strong Religion) (Amharic) (Addis Ababa: Tensae Zagubae Printing Press, 1949 E.C.), pp. 97–98. A similar idea was held by Kidane Wold Kifle who dubbed the writers of *Lefafe* and *Arde'et* 'cheats and impostors'. Kidane Wold Kifle, *Book of Grammar*, p. 570.

15 Tesfa remarked that this prayer, serving as a fortune-bearing charm and blessing one's property, could also protect the bearer from epidemic diseases and ill-intentioned human beings.

16 See also IES, MSS nos. 1056, 1068 and 2151.

17 The word *Asmat* (a plural of the noun ስም or 'name') is believed to be a derivative from a Ge'ez verb ሰየመ, which means 'to give name'.

18 'Malka Giyorgis', 'Malka Ruphael' and 'Mestsehafe Tuladan' are very good examples of magico-religious prayers that contained several talismanic drawings. There is conceivable similarity in the design and supposed importance of the talismanic drawings depicted in these short prayer books. For the whole list of religious and magico-religious texts,

numbering 300, that had been published at Tesfa Gebre Selassie's printing press since its establishment, see Wossen Debebe, *Tesfa Gebre Selassie of Bulga*, pp. 184–193.

19 Oral informant no. 1.

20 Informants have also been critical of Gelahun Abate's published medico-magical text, saying that medical students could not properly utilise it; most of the instructions on the preparation and application of medicaments have been intentionally obscured where, informants alleged, the author did not make clear when and how to collect medicinal herbs, a very challenging area of 'phytotherapic' study. The author, a one-time parliamentarian who claimed that the text was published without his final consent, was blamed for omitting medicinal prescriptions for a complaint such as sexual dysfunction and impotency. Almost all herbal prescriptions in this text have been compounded. In the case of a snake bite, for instance, 46 herbs were needed to prepare the medicine, while other cures were prepared ranging from 4 to more than 20 medicinal plants and herbs. In addition to Ge'ez and Amharic nomenclature, names of plants and herbs have been identified in no less than 11 ethnic languages. Despite its alleged weaknesses, Ahadu's text has been the best medical text ever produced in printed form. See Gelahun Abate, *Book of Herbs: Ethiopian Traditional Medicine* (Amharic) (Addis Ababa: Artistic Printing Press, 1989). Gelahun has been the only cleric–healer praised for the invaluable assistance he provided to the Department of Biology in classifying and registering about 400 Ethiopian herbal drugs. Ministry of Health, *Proceedings of the First National Conference on Ethiopian Traditional Medicine and Healing* (Amharic), Addis Ababa, 27–29 June 1980, p. 72. To date there has been a single printed indigenous medical text for home-based treatment; it is a compilation extracted from very few medical manuscripts, published indigenous and biomedical texts, and journal and newspaper articles, see Bekelech Tolla, *Home-based Therapy: Indigenous Household Treatment with Organic Drugs* (Amharic) (Addis Ababa: Bole Printing Enterprise, 1999 E.C.).

21 Glossaries of Ethiopian plants were published in English by people such as Mooney, Amare, Dawit and Ahadu; and in English and Amharic by Wolde Mikael. See N. F. Mooney, *A Glossary of Ethiopian Plant Names*, (Dublin: Dublin University Press, 1963); Amare Getahun, 'Some Common Medicinal and Poisonous Plants Used in Ethiopian Folk Medicine,' Mimeo. (Addis Ababa University, 1976); Dawit Abebe and Ahadu Ayehu, *Medicinal Plants and Enigmatic Health Practices of Northern Ethiopia*, (Addis Ababa: Berhanena Selam Printing Press, 1993); Azene Bekele Tesemma and Others, *Useful Trees and Shrubs for Ethiopia: Identification, Propagation and Management for Agricultural and Pastoral*

Communities (Nairobi: Swedish International Development Authority, 1993); Walda Mikael Kallacha, *A Glossary of Ethiopian Plant Names*. 4th edition (Addis Ababa: Artistic Printers, 1987); Dawit Abebe and Others, *Medicinal Plants and Other Useful Plants of Ethiopia* (Addis Ababa: Ethiopian Health and Nutrition Research Institute, 2005).

22 Oral informant no. 5.

23 For most cleric–healers, too much reliance on printed texts was no more than restricting oneself to some incomplete or substandard knowledge.

24 *Awda Nagast* (Addis Ababa 1953 E.C.).

25 In 1997 E.C. a certain Gebre Selassie reprinted the 1949 E.C. edition of the *Awda Nagast* without even mentioning the name of Zamanfas Qedus. Gebre Selassie, evading the intellectual property right of the original editor has claimed copyright protection for his illegitimately reproduced text. See Gebre Selassie Berhanu, *Hateta Menafist wa Awda Nagast Kanatalsamu* (Amharic) (Addis Ababa: Aksum Printing Press, 1997 E.C.).

26 An ecclesiastical title bestowed upon a dignitary of the Orthodox Church.

27 Admassu Jembere, *Kokeha Haimanot*, p. 4; a book entitled *Tagsatsena Mekir*, which was considered blasphemous, was the previous work of Zamanfas Qedus. See Zamanfas Qedus Abraha, *Tagsatsena Mekir* (literally 'Reprimand and Advice') (Amharic), 2nd edition (Asmara: Artigraphic Printing Press, 1945 E.C.).

28 Admassu Jembere, *Kokeha Haimanot*, p. 8.

29 See Zamanfas Qedus Abraha, *Hatata Menafist za Awda Nagast*, (Amharic), 2nd edition (Asmara: El Poligraphic Association, 1948 E.C.), pp. 10–11, 13.

30 Quoted in the preface, ibid.

31 His whole argument revolved around the myth of the Fall of Adam and Eve, and the consequential challenges to human beings to live in a world of two contending spirits.

32 Even before the publication of the *Awda Nagast* as a compendium of several divinatory treatises, Tekle Tsadik, a prolific writer of Ethiopian history, severely criticised the divinatory knowledge of cleric–healers. Tekle Tsadik Mekuria, *Human Behavior and Techniques on Social Life* (Amharic) (Addis Ababa: Tensae Zagubae Printing Press, 1951), pp. 136–147. Dr Mérab briefly touched on the issue of consulting astrologers before arranging marriages in the early twentieth century. See Paul Mérab, *Impressions de Ethiopie*, III, p. 80.

33 Alemayehu Moges, 'Traditional Ethiopian Medicine,' *8th International Conference of Ethiopian Studies*. IA, Addis Ababa (1984), p. 134.

34 Alemayehu Moges, 'Traditional Ethiopian Medicine,' p. 134.

35 They argued that publishing such materials was much more damaging than just posing a challenge to healers' monopoly over the written word. Oral informants nos. 2, 30 and 39.

36 Oral informants nos. 2, 30 and 39.

37 The text Griaule published in 1930 was a manuscript Marcel Cohen acquired from a cleric–healer in Gojjam 20 years earlier. See Marcel Griaule, *Le livre de recettes d'un dabtara Abyssin*, (Paris: Institut d'Ethnologie, 1930); Sylvain Grebaut, the editor of *Aethiopica*, a quarterly magazine concerned with the Ge'ez language and literature, edited a number of magico-medical prayers and their French translations in the 1930s. See, for example, 'Prière magique contre la dysenterie'; 'Prière magique contre la pleuresie'; 'Prière contre le peste', *Aethiopica*, 1934; 'Prière pour étre protégé des serpents', *Aethiopica*, 1935; 'Prière magique contre le feu', *Aethiopica*, 1936; 'Prière magique contre la Grele', *Aethiopica*, 1938; *Recueil de texts magiques ethiopiens*, (Paris: Librairie Orientaliste Paul Geuthner, 1939).

38 Haddis Gebre Meskel (ed.), *Book of Medicine: Traditional Ethiopian Medicine*, (London: Haddis Publications, 1988).

39 Stefan Strelcyn, 'Les ecrits medicaux ethiopiens,' *JES*, 3(1) (1965): 82–103.

40 Haddis Gebre Meskel (ed.), *Book of Medicine.*

41 See Ahadu Ayehu, 'Book of Herbs' (Amharic), Unpublished MS (1990).

42 Leul Wolde Ruphael, 'Herbal Medicine' (Amharic), Mimeo (Addis Ababa: National Archives and Libraries, MS no. 492, 1983).

43 *Efran Qalam* constituted pigments of red, blue, black, yellow, brown, light green and dark green.

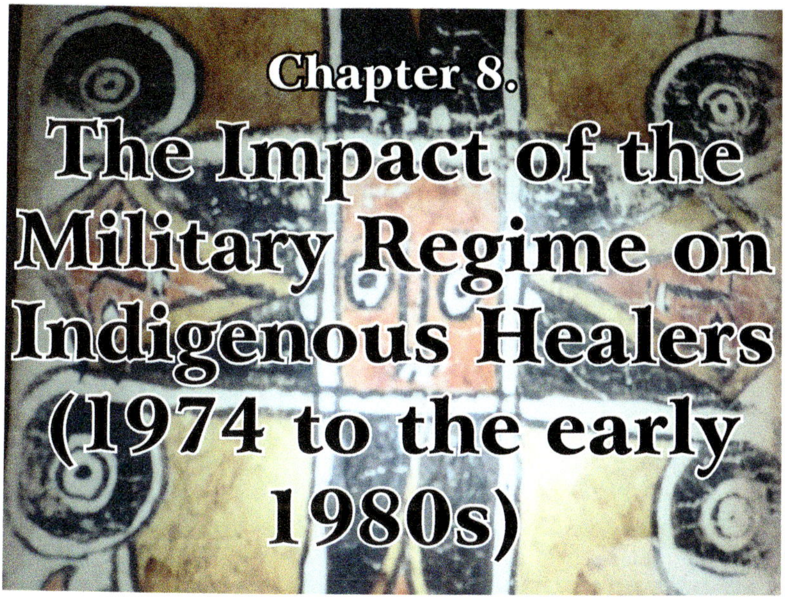

Chapter 8. The Impact of the Military Regime on Indigenous Healers (1974 to the early 1980s)

This chapter examines the condition of indigenous healers during the Darg period with a special focus on church-based medical practitioners. It begins by describing the Marxist military government's anti-religious attacks where indigenous healers, particularly those associated with religious or spiritual healing, became targets of attack by political cadres. The cadres avowed to root out superstitious practices of every stripe and to restructure society. The chapter then looks at how the Darg, recognising the potential value of indigenous medicine, subsequently attempted to integrate it into its primary healthcare system. This effort was inspired, in part, by a wider movement to incorporate indigenous healers into primary health care that was sponsored by the World Health Organization (WHO). By stripping off its religious content, the new regime made futile attempts to reconstitute indigenous healing within a Western biomedical framework. Obviously, these policies alienated church-based healers at the same time as they weakened their position in Ethiopian society. They also made both cleric- and non-cleric–healers suspicious and unsupportive of any state-sponsored initiative towards indigenous medicine; attitudes that have continued up to the present, limiting efforts to develop an integrated health system in Ethiopia today. This chapter examines the fate of indigenous medicine and church-based healers within this general framework during the 1970s and 1980s.

The Darg's Attitude towards Cleric-Healers

Following the popular unrest that swept away the last monarch of the Solomonic Dynasty in 1974, the provisional military government or the Darg (the co-ordinating committee of the Ethiopian Armed Forces and Territorial Army) came to power. The new military government, under increasing pressure from Marxist-oriented intellectuals and the student movement, made it clear that it would follow a socialist path by putting the country's material and non-material resources to the 'communal use of the Ethiopian people'. The government proceeded to take drastic measures against landowners by confiscating agricultural land in rural areas; all urban land and real estate; and financial institutions, large-scale and medium-sized manufacturing, hotel, and business enterprises in urban areas. In the social sphere the military junta made an effort to inculcate the Marxist ideology at the expense of the religious and indigenous belief systems.[1]

The military government, adopting Marx's dictum 'religion is the opium of people', attributed the country's material and cultural backwardness to the people's beliefs in supernatural beings and their adherence to religion. The regime's abhorrence of religious devotions was unequivocally expressed in a confidential communiqué from the Ministry of Information and National Guidance entitled 'Religious Belief is an Enemy to the Revolution'. After making a general assessment of the entrenched position of Orthodox Christianity and Islam among the public and the partnership between the Orthodox Church and the imperial regime, the communiqué called for the immediate eradication of these religious beliefs from Ethiopian soil. To get rid of these beliefs and institutions, the document suggested more than a dozen strategies, including the closure of prominent churches and monasteries, and their subsequent transformation into public art centres, and the collection and removal of all ecclesiastical texts, which the Darg viewed as instrumental in the feudal class exploiting the people.[2]

The Darg repeatedly accused and portrayed the *ancien régime*, or the 'feudo-bourgeois regime', to use their Marxist terminology, as responsible for sponsoring magic and sorcery. The state media proclaimed that 'the emperor and his entourage were fully engaged in this evil [magical] activity'. *Addis Zemen,* the state-run newspaper, claimed that the aristocratic class had tapped the services of astrologers or 'book openers', dream interpreters, magicians and sorcerers in an effort to maintain the feudal system and to exploit the masses. The newspaper went on to say that the imperial regime had even bestowed prestigious titles upon 'magicians' and 'seers'.[3] It also cautioned that magicians and sorcerers who had been largely confined to cheating and exploiting the people had now begun to engage in counter-revolutionary activities, notably providing shelter to reactionary elements and providing hiding places or 'caves' for their weapons and ammunition that would be utilised against the revolution and the 'apostles of the revolution'.[4] Similar allegations were also utilised for closing down evangelical and other non-Orthodox Christian churches.[5]

For their part, many cleric–healer informants alleged that the Darg attacked cleric–healers because some Darg officials, particularly those with a church background, were fearful that the healers' medico-magical knowledge could be employed against them or as an instrument of vengeance in the hands of the ruling classes of the deposed regime. They also claimed that some senior Darg officials utilised the prophetic powers of certain cleric–diviners and healers, and that when these diviners began to make unpromising prophesies about the Darg towards the end of its rule, they executed them.[6]

Whatever the true motivation of the Darg officials may have been, the government launched a series of campaigns against indigenous healers throughout Ethiopia. These campaigns, which were particularly intense between 1976 and 1978, were mostly carried out through state-sponsored, politically affiliated, local-level administrative organs, the infamous *qabale mahbar* (urban dwellers associations) and *gabare mahbar* (farmers associations). During the same period, the revolutionary government initiated a nationwide campaign to eradicate illiteracy, to expand primary health services and to increase basic health education.

Although it is not clear how and when the Darg began its attack on cleric–healers at a national level, the 1975 proclamation of 'Scientific Socialism' or 'Garrison Socialism', as some critics sarcastically called it, may be said to have inaugurated the intimidation of cleric–healers. *Addis Zemen,* as early as September 1975, started publishing news of the detention and confiscation of the property of indigenous medical practitioners. The detention of a 'seer' for being a cheat was a recurrent theme in the newspaper. The early days of the military regime was a very trying time, as many cleric–healers were charged with the offences of practising magico-spiritual healing, and of cheating and exploiting the public. This harassment was part of the Dargs' campaign to re-educate the rural masses.

It was widely reported that participants of the Darg's nation-wide 'Development Through Co-operation' campaign, targeting indigenous health practitioners, irrespective of their title or 'field of specialisation', sent a message to the rural masses that the majority of indigenous healers were impostors and obstacles to the revolutionary changes being introduced in the country.[7] Counting on the support of the state and student campaigners, local-level political and administrative officials detained hundreds of indigenous health practitioners and confiscated their property.[8] Many of the detainees were released after being fined, given some re-education or 'refreshing' political lessons and told to distance themselves from any kind of medical activity in future. A few student campaigners were even killed at the hands of the *qallicha* healers and their retinues.[9]

A medical anthropologist, Mekonnen Bishaw, reviewing the Ethiopian media between 1975 and 1986, asserted that 326 individuals were arrested and charged with practising magic and sorcery, falsely claiming to cure diseases, and for allegedly exploiting the masses. All the accused, apparently found guilty, were fined, sent to prison or subjected to the confiscation of their property.[10] All kinds of household items, such as spears, swords, knives, hammers, umbrellas, snares, beads, drums, rugs, coffee pots and cups, drinking glasses, bells and soap; and magico-medical and religious texts were subject to confiscation. All these objects that were allegedly indispensable to the performance of rituals of magical or spiritual healing sessions were taken away by the notorious local urban and farmers associations. It is worth noting that in spite of the state's repeated efforts to portray healers as politically dangerous elements who had a stake in the previous feudal order, there were only a couple of cases in which firearms were confiscated from indigenous health practitioners. However, healers were arrested for actions that were seen as political. Thus a spiritual healer was incarcerated because he was found guilty of practising magic *and* hanging portraits of the deposed emperor and the royal family on the walls of his residence.[11] 'Healers (particularly spiritual healers) who were caught red-handed in conducting this [magical] activity were forced to march in markets together with their clients and healing objects in order to make them a warning example for others who were conducting such activity,' noted Teshome-Bahiru.[12]

Considering the scale and scope of the campaign, and the apparent exclusion from the media of a string of unreported cases throughout the country, it is likely that Mekonnen's figures underestimate the total number of individuals who were charged for these practices. 'Considerable numbers of healers were put behind bars for conducting false healing which was considered by Marxist cadres as vestiges of the old feudal regime';[13] for example, even after a lapse of two decades, an undergraduate student working on his B.A. thesis found that six out of the dozen indigenous healers he interviewed in Addis Ababa had been harassed by the Darg.[14]

In addition, it is important to recognise that while the number of formal trials of healers in legal courts may have been limited, much of the persecution of healers was carried out extra-legally by urban dwellers and farmers associations. These associations set up their own judicial tribunals or justice committees and dispensed 'instant', often iniquitous, judgments on the accused. The accused were penalised with hard cash penalties, imprisonment or both.[15]

One of the primary purposes of the attacks on healers was the confiscation of religious texts. In some cases, written magico-medical materials were clearly stated in the lists of confiscated items, while in many other cases, the record only refers to 'items related to magical activity and sorcery have been confiscated'. Such items, no doubt, included a good number of written magico-medical texts.[16]

To hunt down written magico-medical texts, a committee of local administrative and political cadres repeatedly ransacked healers' houses; and whenever this committee found written materials, it simply tore them into pieces, burnt them on the spot or took them to be used later as evidences against cleric–healers.[17] After being detained, a cleric–healer was asked to hand over his medico-magical texts, but he would be set free if no medico-magical text was found in his house during the *asesa* (searching operation). Recalling the trauma he had gone through, a cleric–healer stated, 'If they [state agents] had found the medico-magical text in my house, I could have been killed.'[18] Knowing that the cadres would someday come to his house in search of written materials, he hid his treasured text of more than four hundred parchment vellums, which he had acquired and copied in the mid-1930s from a certain *alaqa* in Gondar, in exchange for a rifle.[19] It would have been 'a great loss for me and my career had my incarcerators found the text in my house and confiscated it,' he added. It was a terrible tragedy, informants reminisced, that inestimable quantities of medical texts were 'looted or vanished before our eyes'.[20] Another informant witnessed a house-to-house search carried out by the security forces looking for illegal arms and written materials of reactionary content. The searchers had entered his father's house and confiscated a patchwork of purely religious manuscripts, some of which were made of horse skin, which his cleric father had collected during his life-long ecclesiastical service. The manuscripts were lost forever. Even many under-age children who possessed inherited medico-magical texts of their parents were targeted. However, it should be noted that many cleric–healers living in relatively remote rural localities and in some bigger towns did not experience these problems, and their medico-magical texts were neither confiscated nor destroyed.[21]

Some cleric–healers, being aware of the prevailing situation and warned about the destructive actions of the political agents in other places, succeeded in saving their medical texts from destruction or confiscation. Preservation of medico-magical texts was partly possible by locking them in iron boxes and burying them in the ground or sending them to relatives living in far-off places.[22] Thus, one informant remembered: 'Based on the information they got from my previous student, the cadres ransacked my house more than a couple of times without search warrants, but I pre-empted them by burying all my precious medico-magical texts beneath the floor of my house using a new earthenware pot from which I retrieved them after the removal from power of the Darg.'[23] Similarly, a herbalist was forced to bury his medical text which he bought from an illiterate person who had obtained it through inheritance, because, as he put it, 'I took this precautionary measure because the spirit of the time was unfavourable to all indigenous health practitioners, including herbalists; and to be frank, everyone was on edge since possession of a medical text was just enough to be arrested.'[24]

Regrettably, however, medico-magical texts that were not properly buried or concealed were found partially or wholly spoilt when retrieved after two or more years.[25] A cleric–healer 'felt a wave of fury running through him' when he found his medico-magical texts entirely spoilt as he dug them out from a nearby cave after a couple of years. He observed: 'The only thing I benefited from this sorry state of affair was that the authorities at that time could not find any evidence to accuse me or put me in prison.'[26]

Cleric– and secular healers were also forced to hand over specimens of their herbal medicines to individuals from the Ministry of Health; an act that was viewed by healers as 'blatant robbery'.[27] 'I was put in jail while returning home from my journey to Matakal and Assosa in search of medicinal plants, and the authorities released me when they did not find any written medico-magical texts with me, and still, I was forced to hand over all the medicinal plants I kept in my bag,'[28] a cleric–healer noted.

A few healers took direct actions against the cadres who searched their premises for manuscripts. In one case, a cleric–healer cast a magic spell called *andereb* against a local cadre, who had assaulted the cleric for no tangible reason. The cadre, realising the futility of seeking other healers to assist him, and being frantic to free himself from the influence of the spell, bargained with the healer who had put the hex on him. Before revoking his magic spell, the cleric told the cadre to be mindful of the futility of counting on Marxism; a hollow ideology that could not protect him from similar incidents in future, and advised him to abstain from such provocative deeds.[29]

In the end, the activities of the political cadres resulted in the destruction of highly treasured and historically valuable medico-magical materials, which should have been given special care and preservation. Some informants compared the sacking of religious texts to what had occurred during 'the destructive Moslem–Christian conflicts of the sixteenth century'.[30] Dawit and Ahadu claimed that the Darg, in its effort to destroy the church and the Orthodox faith 'inflicted probably as much damage as the invading [British] forces [that stormed Maqdala in the nineteenth century] to medico-religious literature'.[31] Such comparisons and inferences may not, in fact, do justice to the destruction imposed by the Darg, for many of the manuscripts looted by the British have been preserved in England, while the ambit of destruction on the country's literary heritage by the Darg was enormous, irretrievable and thus far more serious than that caused by the British invaders.[32]

Others have compared the Darg's persecution of indigenous healers to the efforts of Emperor Yohannes IV (1872–1889),[33] who tried to destroy traditional practices and force the conversion of Ethiopian Muslims to Orthodox Christianity.[34]

Reconstituting Indigenous Healing Within 'Scientific Medicine'

While the Darg and its political cadres attacked practitioners of traditional medicine for a range of political and ideological reasons, the regime claimed that it was not opposed to indigenous medicine, as such, but believed that it needed to be made more scientific and accessible to the people. To this end, traditional medicine needed to be stripped of its 'superstitious roots', making its vast knowledge accessible for medical investigation and use. From this perspective, the regime's attacks on healers and confiscation of medical texts can be seen as an initial destructive salvo aimed at dislodging indigenous medicine from its religious base. Claiming to have achieved this goal, the regime turned fitfully to reconstituting indigenous medicine under a new scientific guise. Unfortunately, the Darg's lack of control over its overly enthusiastic cadres and its association of healers with political opposition resulted in the destruction of many texts that might have contributed to their quest for usable indigenous medicines.

After a lapse of years of uncertainty, confusion and destruction, the Ministry of Public Health began to talk about the urgent need to do something about indigenous medicine and healing. The first step was taken in February 1977 when a 'permanent committee' of scholars was established with a view to conducting research on indigenous medicine and using its results to the benefit of the broad masses. The committee acknowledged, though belatedly, that written medical and magical texts known by a generic name *Etse Dabdabe* ('Book of Herbs', constituting often varied forms of magico-medical texts) and *Asmat* ('Secret Names' or, better yet, 'Magic Prayers') were potential sources of future research. It also stated that most of these texts were kept in churches, mosques, police stations, and in urban dwellers' and peasant associations.[35] Those in the possession of the police and peasant associations had been confiscated from cleric–healers. Many others, as indicated, had been destroyed. Had the committee's commitment to preserving indigenous medical knowledge been rightfully and genuinely carried out, this destruction could have been stymied and the country's cultural legacy preserved.

Unfortunately, the committee's plan to research and compile a nation-wide inventory of the confiscated written medico-magical texts did not materialise.[36] Yet, the Darg's acknowledgement that indigenous medicine had value, opened up space for indigenous healers to begin reasserting themselves within the medical landscape, albeit half-heartedly, by organising professional associations.

Towards the end of the 1950s, a few indigenous health practitioners had begun to come together for the first time to form a professional association in Addis Ababa, However, this association did not last long, primarily because there was no harmony among practitioners and, secondly, because it did not obtain the support of the imperial government, which was not gracious to all labour organisations and professional associations. As a result, practitioners continued to carry on their duties independently of one another; a situation that continued until the popular uprising in the mid-1970s.[37]

With the overthrow of the imperial government and the issuance, in 1975, of the labour proclamation, labour unions and professional associations were theoretically able to organise.[38] The new 'freedom' to form independent professional associations was also extended to indigenous medical practitioners. However, the reality on the ground was quite different due partly to unfavourable political circumstances; indigenous healers up to 1976/77 made little progress in organising their associations.[39]

One of the major obstacles to the creation of healers association was the Darg's insistence that responsibility for establishing these associations be entrusted to 'the Coordinating Office for Traditional Medicine and Healing', an office that came into being in 1975 within the Ministry of Health, rather than to healers themselves. This office, in turn, delegated its responsibility to provincial health departments, which were charged with[40] registering indigenous healers, organising healers associations and overseeing their activities in their respective provinces. The local health departments, however, being more interested in controlling indigenous health practitioners than in mobilising them to the envisaged goal, failed to follow through on their responsibilities. Relations between the health departments and local indigenous healers were, in fact, strained. Health department officials were sceptical about the value of indigenous medicine, and the healers, who had gone through some dreadful experiences during the early period of the Darg rule, did not trust the health departments. Indigenous health practitioners did not see any tangible reason to have faith in health departments, which they perceived as instruments of an unpredictable state, a state that had been bent on destroying the country's literary and medical heritages.

Despite their general apathy towards the Ministry of Public Health, indigenous healers in the provinces had no choice but to comply with the call for registration by the health departments; and many healers felt compelled to register as members of the politically monitored professional associations. No less critical, indigenous healers joined these associations because they did not want to be labelled as traitors, reactionaries or enemies of the revolution. It should be noted that, in line with the ministry's effort to separate indigenous medicine from its religious roots, spiritual and cleric–healers were not formally invited to become members. As a result, indigenous practitioners whose healing strategies constituted predominantly herbal medicine became favoured and principal members of these associations. Yet the association membership lists reveal the names of a number of Christian and Muslim cleric–healers, suggesting that the ministry was unable to separate out religious-based healing completely.

The coordinating office made it clear that its main objective was to help the country become self-reliant in medicine, and to free itself from the economic domination and cultural influence of Western imperialist nations. In order to achieve this goal, indigenous health practitioners had to adopt biomedical or 'scientific' diagnostic and treatment methods in place of their timeworn diagnostic and therapeutic strategies. The office noted further that this transformation would give indigenous practitioners the liberty to render efficient services and to work towards integrating indigenous medicine into the Western medical system. The goal was to make indigenous medicine an appendage to Western-style health care and create a cadre of traditional medical practitioners who would co-operate with practitioners of biomedicine. Like efforts at integration in other parts of the world, integration essentially meant, on the one hand, stripping away scientifically validated indigenous medicines from the complex diagnostic and therapeutic systems in which they were situated, while, on the other, allocating ailments that were thought to be idiopathic and beyond the reach of Western biomedicine, to indigenous healers.[41] This definition of traditional medical practitioners, combined with the regime's general attack on religious practices, meant that the system favoured herbalists and other non-cleric–healers over church-based healers.

The goal of integrating indigenous and Western medicine had been repeatedly proposed, beginning with Menelik's pragmatic efforts. The integration effort of the 1950s has been a missed opportunity. In an Amharic work of fiction of the early 1960s entitled *Traditional Medicine by Indigenous Scholars*,[42] the author, describing poignantly the ways in which traditional medicine was functioning, and its potential values to the people and the country, proposed a strategy for putting these possibilities into practice. He called upon indigenous practitioners, notably cleric–healers and Ethiopian students learning Western medicine in Europe, to come together and establish healthcare facilities that would provide people with indigenous and biomedical services simultaneously. The writer believed fervently that the mistrust between practitioners of the two medical systems would be alleviated by encouraging a dialogue that could eventually lead to their integration.[43] The idea of co-operation between the allopathic and indigenous medicine during the Darg era was thus a continuation of a nationalist effort that had a long history in Ethiopia. Yet for most of this period, practitioners of indigenous medicine and Western medicine were more likely to see themselves as rivals in a medical marketplace than as partners in a common medical system; a scheme that required both groups of practitioners to keep their pledge and serve the people honestly and diligently.

The Darg's rhetorical embraced of the notion of integration was also encouraged by the WHO, of which Ethiopia was a member, and which in the late 1970s adopted integration as one of its official guidelines. With the intention of restructuring the health needs of the developing world, the WHO recommended increased research into herbal and magico-religious cures of indigenous health practitioners, and emphasised the need to establish national healers associations that would help healers realise their strength. The WHO's strategy also encouraged 'frequent discussions among all the experts of both the traditional and allopathic systems [so as] . . . to create a climate for promoting a synthesis of the best of all systems'.[44] In order to execute this, a vibrant body or system had to be put in place to win the trust of indigenous practitioner and bring them into close dialogue with practitioners of Western biomedicine.

Such a goal was difficult to achieve in Ethiopia for two reasons. First, the state failed to create the necessary organisation to institute co-operation among different groups of healers. Second, indigenous healers were mistrustful of the state's efforts in the light of the earlier, and in some cases ongoing, unco-operative and/or destructive attitude of Western health practitioners towards indigenous healers. This mistrust was only increased by the ways in which the Ministry of Health went about enlisting or, more accurately, demanding the co-operation of healers.

Following the establishment of healers associations, the ministry compelled indigenous healers to hand over specimens of their herbal medicines to the health departments, claiming that they would be used for future scientific investigations.[45] Healers resented this use of coercion by the Mengistu government to extract ethno-botanical knowledge from herbalists and were suspicious of the government's motives.[46]

This combination of mistrust and resentment led many healers simply to provide the health departments with specimens of common botanical remedies having little medicinal value. Alemayehu, a lecturer in the language department at Addis Ababa University since the early 1960s and a full-time cleric–healer after his retirement in 1981/82, has been quoted as saying, 'The deceivers were deceived and the cheats were cheated, in between them [sic] true wisdom was buried forever.'[47] The kind of relationship cleric–healers maintained with the Ministry of Public Health during the Darg may be termed a 'cat-and-mouse game' where practitioners were increasingly forced to go underground[48] and to reject a strategy of 'creative accommodation'[49] with institutions that hyped and endorsed the supremacy of Western medicine over indigenous medicine.

Though the military regime claimed to have demonstrated an unusually avant-garde stand towards indigenous medicine and healing, it dismissed the value of church-based (or other streams of spiritual healers) in favour of lay herbalists, traditional birth attendants and bone-setters. The Darg government viewed 'men of letters' (cleric–healers) as fans or stooges of the previous regime, and adopted an officially discriminatory stance against them. This dismissal of church-based healing was in line with its broader attack on anything Orthodox or religious.[50] This policy discounted the value to the country's literary healing tradition, as well as the important role that cleric–healers played in the medical marketplace.

The Darg and the Training of Cleric–healers

Church-based healers viewed the Darg's destructive policies as responsible not only for the declining importance of church-based medicine, but also for disrupting the training of a new generation of cleric–healers in the country. The ability of church healers to train students was threatened by the Darg's attack on the economic foundations of the Orthodox Church, and by its repression of church-based healers and confiscation of their medical texts.

The proclamations in 1975 of 'Public Ownership of Rural Lands and Extra Houses in Urban Areas' severely undermined the economic foundation of the church and its nearly 200 000 priests and church workers.[51] Throughout its existence, the Orthodox Church had appropriated vast tracts of land, along with thousands of tenants who worked these lands. This provided the church with massive amounts of wealth in the form of land taxes. The church's longstanding rights to these taxes were embodied in Article 2 of the 1942 proclamation related to church lands, which read:

> Those who own landed properties . . . in the capacity of '*Alaqa*', or '*Gebez*', 'Priest', 'Deacon', '*Debtara*' or holder of any other different office of this nature by which the Church is served, are to pay money to the church, while the land and fiefs are in their possession, according to the rate of tax assessed by the government.[52]

After the confiscation of its urban properties and rural agricultural lands in 1975,[53] the Orthodox Church became almost entirely dependent on the financial and material contributions of its members. Lacking the support of the revolutionary government, which was intent on down-grading the role of Christianity in Ethiopian society and suppressing religious education, the church had serious difficulty maintaining its schools[54] estimated to be around 8 000, with the capacity to accommodate close to 200 000 students.[55] The difficulty in eking out a livelihood with only the contributions of the laity compelled many church scholars and cleric–healers to migrate to the cities in search of employment in urban churches. Those who opted not to migrate to the urban centres had to endure a variety of problems, including lack of basic necessities.

The combination of economic hardship and religious suppression, which included the persecution of cleric–healers and confiscation of medical texts, described above, made it hard for the church to carry out its spiritual duties or to attract and retain learned clerics and religious students as well. In addition, individual cleric teachers found it difficult and even dangerous to carry out their medico-magical instructions; and those who did, needed to observe extreme care and vigilance. What should be stressed here is that during the early days of the Darg, the teaching–learning process of church-based medicine was subject to new levels of secrecy, previously unknown. The spirit of insecurity and suspicion besetting both teachers and students was so strong that many cleric–healer–teachers discontinued teaching medico-magical subjects altogether.

Despite these challenges, teaching church-based medicine continued, albeit in an attenuated state. A few intrepid cleric–healers resolved to pass on the healing arts to their disciples. By doing so they hoped to ensure the survival of a limited amount of church-based medical knowledge. However, this had to be done with extreme care and secrecy. As a result, the nature of the educational process was compromised. Unlike previous times, cleric teachers during the Darg were hesitant to use their medico-magical manuscripts as instructional materials for their students, lest they be confiscated. Informants unanimously stressed that under these conditions exchanging medico-magical information was not easy. The amount of medico-magical knowledge imparted to medical students during the Darg was dismayingly negligible. In addition, the possibility of transmitting distorted information that could be dangerous was high.

The limited possibilities for carrying out formal education meant that the quality and reputation of church healing suffered, as poorly trained students portrayed themselves as qualified cleric–healers. This was a serious setback for church-based medicine, and it heralded an epoch of decline that would not be reversed even after the downfall of the military rule. In the end, the Darg's destructive attitude towards church-based healing and support of non-literate healers who could not read or write Ge'ez magico-medical texts, resulted in the demoralisation of cleric–healers, speeded up the decline of their valuable medical profession, and prevented the transmission of their medical knowledge to a new generation of healers.[56]

The Report of the First National Conference on indigenous medicine, organised by the state in 1980, provided ample evidence of the extent to which cleric healing had been marginalised under the Darg.[57] The conference's proposals for the creation of healers associations left little room for church-based healing. Instead, healers associations were supposed to be based on socialist principles with a view to protecting healers' interests and helping them serve the broad masses accordingly.[58] Healers associations were also depicted as platforms for practitioners to get to know one another and to differentiate the genuine from the impostor; to overcome the problem of secrecy with which indigenous medicine and healing were inherently associated; to record and put a stop to the disappearance of medical information transmitted orally from the previous generation; and, finally, to enable the country to have a national herbal pharmacopoeia.[59] No mention was made of the value of magico-religious/magico-medical texts and the healing modalities of church-based healers; a conflicting position to one of the WHO's proposals.

In summary, denigrating cleric–healers and destroying Ethiopia's literary medical heritage was the hallmark of the military regime. The Darg inflicted irreparable damage on church-based medicine at the same time that it cynically praised the value of 'indigenous medicine'. No wonder that its insincerity further undermined the little positive achievement to its credit. It also prevented the perpetuation of church-based healing through an unbroken chain of recruitment and training of cleric–healers, a situation that lingers even today. More importantly, the Darg's misguided efforts to define and regulate indigenous medical practices greatly contributed to the distortion of church-affiliated medico-magical wisdom; a vital condition to the appearance of a substantial number of untrained or fraudulent healers. 'In the country where the unemployment rate is extremely high,' remarked Teshome, 'indulging oneself in the healing profession became a source of income for a considerable section of the population in Addis Ababa.'[60] In the end, one cannot even say that the government merely tried and, ultimately failed, to promote indigenous medicine or to make peace with healers. The injudicious attitude of the Darg discouraged indigenous medical practitioners from taking any active part in efforts to integrate them into the country's health system. Viewed in this light, it is unsurprising that the knowledge imbedded in indigenous medical texts and the ability to deploy it properly is in danger of disappearing. A similar logic can be applied to the incapacity of indigenous healers to divulge the curing potential ascribed to their magico-religious/magico-medical healing techniques.

Figure 19: A talismanic drawing for attracting good fortune

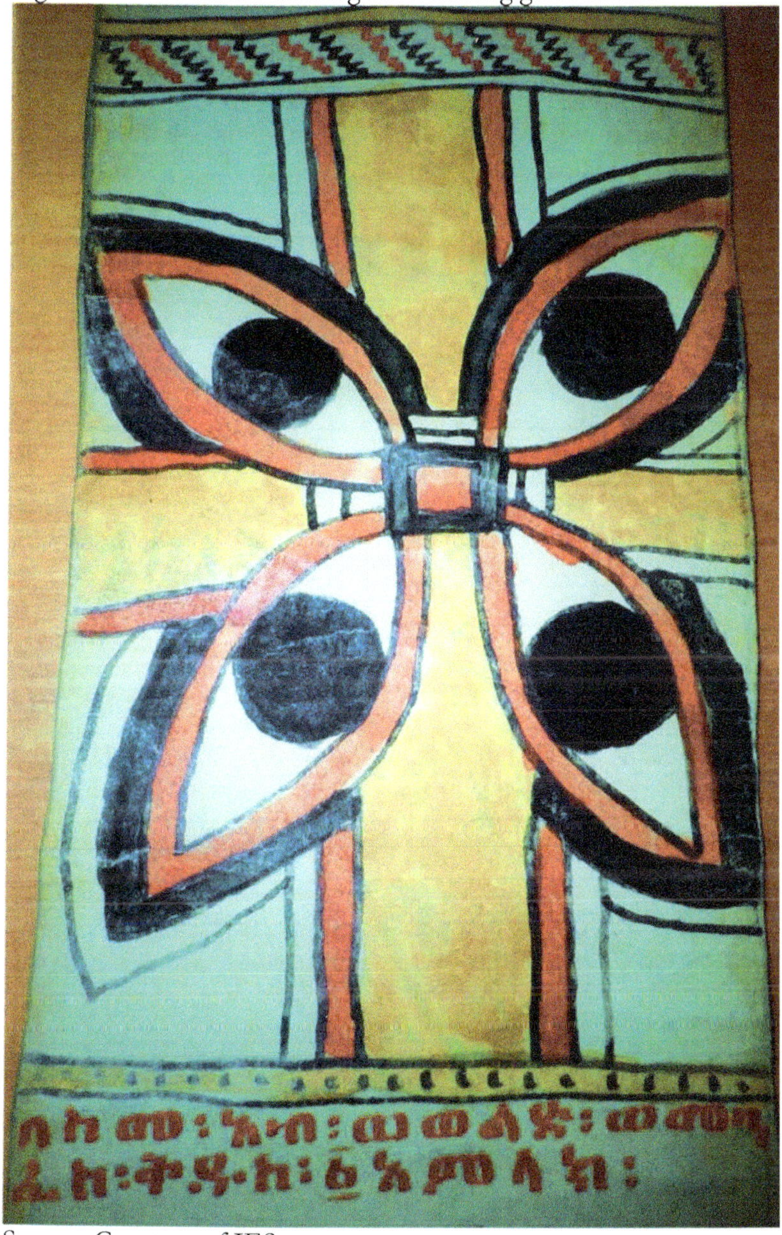

Source: Courtesy of IES

Figure 20: A magical amulet against miscarriage (?)

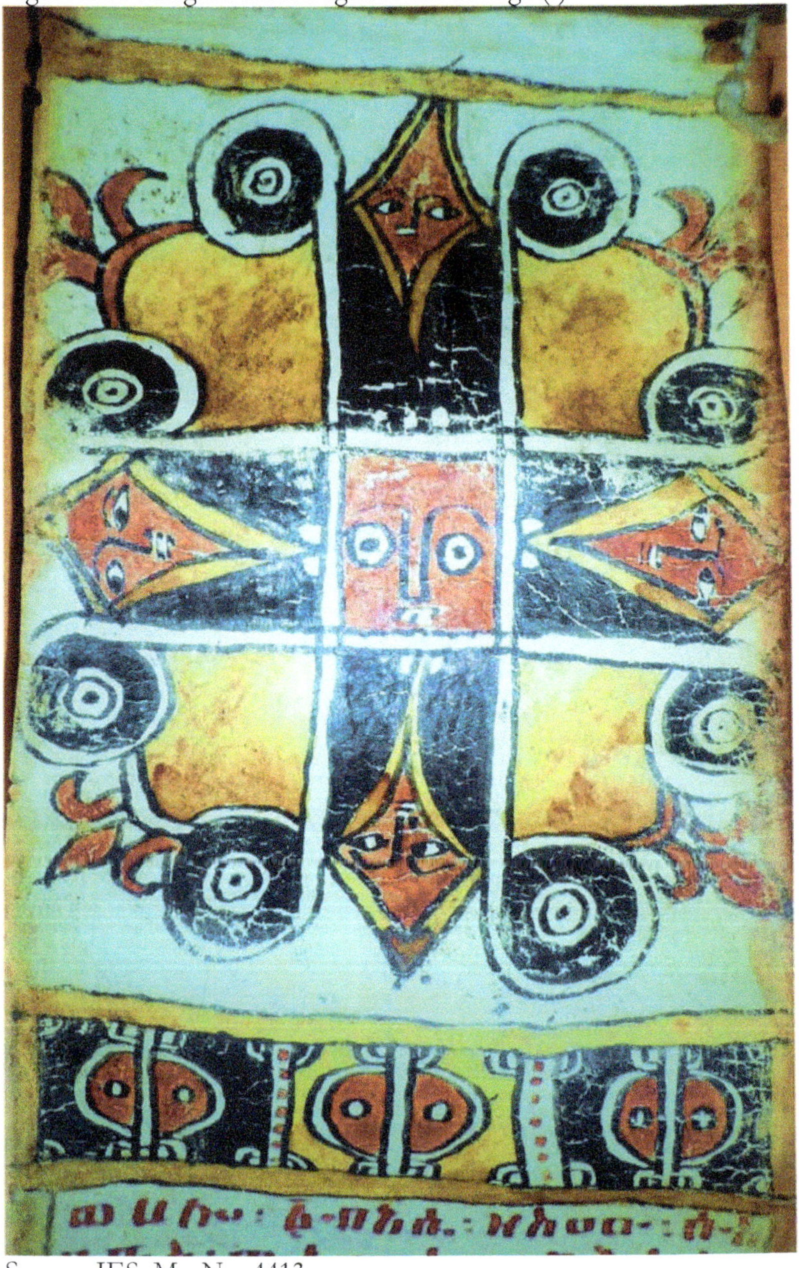

Source: IES, Ms. No. 4413

Notes

1 Fikre Selassie Wogderes, *We and the Revolution.* (Amharic) (Addis Ababa: Tsehay Printing Press, 2006 E.C.), pp. 155–185.

2 Ministry of Information and National Guidance, a communiqué entitled 'Religious Belief is an Enemy to the Revolution', n.d.

3 Bestowing honourable titles on spiritual healers was one of the most sporadic allegations against the deposed emperor. See, for example, Fantahun Engeda, *Major Political Problems and Struggles During Haile Selassie's Administration as Learned from the Biography of the Emperor's Close Associates* (Amharic) (Addis Ababa: Berhanena Selam Printing Press, 1997 E.C.), p. 278.

4 *Addis Zemen*, 20 October 1976.

5 Oyvind Eide, *Revolution and Religion in Ethiopia*, (Oxford: James Currey, 2000), pp. 172, 205.

6 Tilahun Berhane Selassie, *Twentieth Century Ethiopia*, volume 1 (Amharic) (Addis Ababa: Artistic Printing Press, 1998 E.C.), p. 400.

7 Oral informants nos. 11, 27, 30 and 37.

8 Fikre Selassie Wogderes, *We and the Revolution* (Amharic) (Addis Ababa: Tsehay Printing Press, 2006 E.C., pp. 162–164.

9 Ibid.

10 Mekonnen Bishaw, 'Promoting Traditional Medicine in Ethiopia', *Social Science and Medicine* 33(2) (1991): 198–199.

11 *Addis Zemen*, 2 October 1978.

12 Wondwosen Teshome-Bahiru, 'Impacts of Urbanisation on the Traditional Medicine of Ethiopia', *Anthropologist* 8(1) (2005): p. 45.

13 Ibid.

14 Biniam Weldegebreil, 'Traditional Medicine Practitioners of Addis Ababa: A Historical Account from Imperial Times to the Present,' unpublished B.A. thesis (Addis Ababa University, History, 1998), p. 14.

15 Healers had to endure one to six months of incarceration and a fine ranging between 50 and 300 birr. In a related case, 16 421.25 birr was confiscated from a single healer, and the confiscated money, together with other household items, was declared public property. *Addis Zemen*, 2 June 1977.

16 In one case, for instance, 13 Arabic texts were confiscated from a woman healer. *Addis Zemen*, 22 December 1976.

17 Oral informants nos. 11, 22, 24, 27 and 30.

18 Oral informant no. 24.

19 Oral informant no. 27. The informant underscored that his magico-medical text was entirely prepared out of horse skin.

20 Unlike the most common manuscripts made out of sheep skin (on account of their yellowish tinge, they were often used for non-religious texts), goat, ox, and cow skins, some of the destroyed parchment texts were allegedly produced from the skins of horses, donkeys and from wild animals such as bushbuck, antelope and bush duiker. Owing to their whiteness, the skins of goats and antelopes were the most preferred ones for religious books.

21 Oral informants nos. 18 and 31.

22 Oral informants nos. 22 and 27.

23 Oral informant no. 35.

24 Oral informant no. 16.

25 Oral informants nos. 11 and 20.

26 Oral informant no. 37.

27 Oral informant no. 11.

28 Oral informant no. 19.

29 Oral informant no. 58.

30 Oral informant no. 18.

31 Dawit Abebe and Ahadu Ayehu, *Medicinal Plants and Enigmatic Health Practices of Northern Ethiopia* (Addis Ababa: Berhanena Salam Printing Press, 1993), p. 3.

32 To uproot the ideology of the 'old feudo-bourgeois order' and to inculcate the political dogma of the 'new political order', the military regime went to the extent of burning books held in schools and libraries.

33 Jacques Mercier, *Asres: Le magicien ethiopien* (Paris: Jean-Claude Lattes, 1988), p. 13; Mercier wrote that '*l'atmosphere politique avant 1985 n'etat pas favorable aux medicins traditionels*', ibid.

34 Bahru, quoting Gebre Hiywot Baykedagne, see Bahru Zewde, *Pioneers of Change in Ethiopia: Reformist Intellectuals of the Early Twentieth Century* (Addis Ababa: Addis Ababa University Press, 2002), p. 153.

35 *Addis Zemen*, 3 February 1977.

36 Ibid.

37 Biniam Weldegebreil, 'Traditional Medicine Practitioners of Addis Ababa', p. 34.

38 Ethiopian Government, Labor Proclamation, *Negarit Gazeta*, Proclamation no. 158, 1975.

39 The already established associations made only a few steps forward. In this connection, other than the two healers associations that existed in name in the provinces of Tigray and Bale, associations in other provinces did not survive the Darg period. At a conference held in Addis Ababa in August 1980, a coordinating committee was set up to

organise a national healers association, but due to its weakened position, the committee itself was destined to disintegrate.

40 This department was assisted by the National Advisory Committee constituting 12 educational, research and professional associations. This advisory committee was intended to strengthen the ad hoc committee of physicians established in 1976.

41 See, for example, Stacy Pigg's article on the implementation of an integrated health system in Nepal, 'Acronyms and Effacement: Traditional Medical Practitioners (TMP) in International Health Development', *Social Science and Medicine*, 41 (1995): pp. 47–68

42 Sahle Mikael Wolde Selassie, 'Traditional Medicine by Indigenous Scholars' (Amharic) (Addis Ababa: Tensae Zagubae Printing Press, 1956 E.C.).

43 See, Sahle Mikael Wolde Selassie, *Traditional Medicine by Indigenous Scholars*.

44 'Report of the Consultation on Approaches for Policy Development for Traditional Health Practitioners, Including Traditional Birth Attendants' (Geneva: WHO 1985), p. 37; see also World Health Organization, *Primary Health Care: Report of the International Care*, Alma-Ata, USSR (Geneva: WHO, 1978).

45 As in the 1940s and 1950s, the notion of obtaining lists of healers' medicine remained the unchanged motto of the Ministry of Health; see, for example, Ministry of Health, file no. ገሁ 23/45/13, 5 April 1989.

46 Norbert Vecchiato, 'Traditional Medicine,' In the *Ecology of Health and Disease*, edited by Helmut Kloos and Zein Ahmed Zein (Colorado: Westview Press, 1993), p. 174. There is an abundant literature on the efforts to integrate indigenous health practices, including traditional midwifery, with the biomedical system. See, for example, Mekonnen Bishaw, 'Attitudes of Modern and Traditional Medical Practitioners towards Co-operation,' *Ethiopian Medical Journal*, 28 (1990); Mekonnen Bishaw, 'Integrating Indigenous and Cosmopolitan Medicine in Ethiopia,' unpublished Ph.D. dissertation (Southern Illinois University, 1988).

47 Alemayehu Moges, 'Traditional Ethiopian Medicine,' *8th International Conference of Ethiopian Studies*, VI, Addis Ababa, 1984, p. 133.

48 Norbert Vecchiato, 'Traditional Medicine,' *Ecology of Health and Disease*, p. 157.

49 Diana Zeller, 'Traditional and Western Medicine in Buganda: Coexistence and Complement', *Rural Africana*, 26 (1974/5): pp. 91–103.

50 The Darg succeeded in executing its anti-religious policy through 'careful elimination of potentially critical elements' and controlling the

central administration of the Ethiopian Orthodox Church. See Oyvind Eide, *Revolution and Religion in Ethiopia*, pp. 173–174.

51 Oyvind Eide, *Revolution and Religion in Ethiopia*, p. 29; according to the 1970 statistics of the Orthodox Church, the number of clergy was 191 209, of which 48 269 were *dabtara*. See *The Ethiopian Orthodox Church: A Panorama of History and Spiritual Life* (Addis Ababa: A Publication of the EOC, 1997), p. 125.

52 Imperial Ethiopian Government, *Negarit Gazeta*, 'Regulation for the Administration of the Church', November 1942.

53 The vast tracts of land that the church owned were mostly of gifts of the crown, the nobility and rich landowners.

54 Bitew Kassaw, 'Migration of Clergymen from Rural Areas to the Cities: The Case in Addis', unpublished B.Th. thesis, (Holy Trinity Theological College, 2001).

55 Oyvind Eide, *Revolution and Religion*, p. 168.

56 Oral informants nos. 1 and 2.

57 Ministry of Health, *Proceedings of the First National Conference on Ethiopian Traditional Medicine and Healing* (Amharic), Addis Ababa, 27–29 June 1980.

58 Though the 1948 proclamation was not formally abrogated or substituted with a new legal code, all work licences issued by the previous government were declared null and void; and, in future, stated the Minister of Public Health, indigenous practitioners would have new permission papers to verify their registration; and the previous ten years requirement was theoretically replaced with a minimum of five years' work experience. For a sample of the draft registration format, see Ministry of Health, *Proceedings of the First National Conference*, pp. 103–108, also pp. 19–23.

59 Ibid, pp. 82–83.

60 Wondwosen Teshome-Bahiru, 'Impacts of Urbanisation', p. 45.

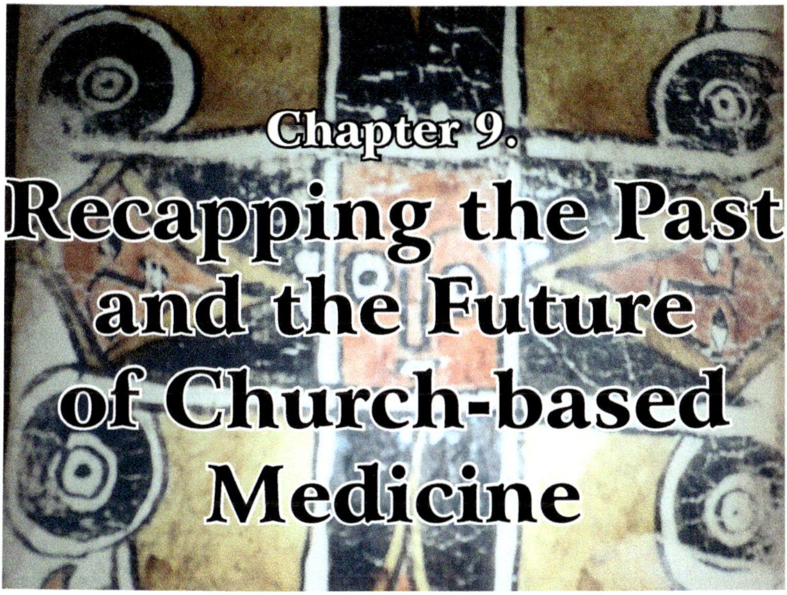

Chapter 9.

Recapping the Past and the Future of Church-based Medicine

In the early twentieth century church-based healers constituted a sizeable number of literate health practitioners in the Amhara region of Ethiopia. They provided their medico-magical services to a cross-section of the region's population. However, the expansion of Western biomedicine and education posed a formidable challenge to the nearly monopolistic position of cleric–healers. They had to devise strategies to ensure their survival in the changing society where the state was bent on structuring the country's healthcare system along biomedical lines. Cleric–healers had to find ways to work in a pluralistic medical environment.

Until the middle of the 1930s, church-based healers were able to sustain their medical dominance, as Western biomedicine made only limited inroads. Under the Italians, however, attacks on healers for their alleged involvement in political resistance, combined with an expansion of biomedical services, began to undermine this dominance.

With the restoration of the imperial regime, the position of church-based healers was further eroded. Though the indigenous therapeutic system was accorded legal recognition, the place of church-based healers was not clearly delineated; and their position was further undermined by the rapid expansion of Western education and literacy, and the growth of printing technology. The imperial government also expanded biomedical services though, as has been pointed out, the provision of services was handicapped by an inefficient bureaucracy. Finally, the emergence of new forms of healing, including hybrid healers and 'injectionists', expanded the therapeutic options available to Ethiopian, further challenging the position of cleric healers.

Under the military government that took control of the country in 1974, church-based healers faced new challenges. The Darg's efforts to eliminate religion, including forms of healing that were based on religious beliefs, put church-based medicine in a state of confusion, and disrupted the production of learned healers. It also reduced the importance of church schools and the attraction of students to these institutions of learning. However, the deterioration of the public health system and the adoption of the WHO's 1978 Primary Healthcare Strategy, persuaded the military government to soften its hostile attitude towards indigenous healers. In acknowledging the value of indigenous medical knowledge, however, the Darg emphasised what it saw as is practical elements, focusing primarily on herbal remedies. At the same time, it largely rejected the value of spiritual healing and the religious aspects of church-based medicine. It focused mostly on the training of traditional birth attendants, and excluded other indigenous healers from taking part in the primary health-care training programmes. While it created a Coordinating Office for Traditional Medicine, and organised a limited number of seminars and workshops on indigenous medicine, these activities did little to overcome the suspicion that healers had of a government that had earlier attempted to eliminate their practices.

While indigenous healers faced administrative actions that threatened their ability to practise openly, the Haile Selassie period represented an era of relative openness and freedom to indigenous medical practitioners, including church-based healers, when compared to the Italian era and the post-Haile Selassie period. And yet, the authority of church-based healing began to be seriously undermined by the rapid expansion of Western education, and the growth of printing and literacy during the same period.

The government that succeeded the military regime in 1991 incorporated traditional medicine in its health policy. The 1993 health policy speaks to the need to develop traditional medicine, including the adoption of regulations and registration of healers, and its gradual integration into the biomedical system. However, little has been accomplished so far; and at present there are no registered or licensed healers or guidelines and training programmes for them.

The efforts of successive Ethiopian governments to deal with indigenous healers have failed to achieve an effective integration of indigenous healing practices and Western biomedicine. To the contrary, repeated attacks on healers, combined with misguided efforts to define and regulate indigenous medical practices, have discouraged healers from participating in efforts to integrate them into the country's health system. At the same time, since the Italian era, state policies have undermined the practice of church-based healing that had once dominated the medical marketplace among the Amhara, and prevented the training of new generations of cleric healers. The knowledge imbedded in esoteric magico-medical texts and the ability to deploy it properly is in danger of disappearing.

To save indigenous medicine from vanishing, there must be a strong and positive attitude, and sense of direction and purpose on the part of both indigenous health practitioners and state officials to finding ways to preserve, value and utilise the rich body of indigenous medical knowledge that is rapidly disappearing. It requires the creation of new institutions that will take this goal seriously and create opportunities to explore opportunities for integrating indigenous therapies into the Ethiopia's health system. Unlike the committee created in the 1950s for this purpose, new institutions must purposely engage with indigenous healers.

Most cleric–healers today decry the absence of individuals or organisations with a commitment to learning, evaluating and preserving the indigenous medico-magical lore. They are extremely passionate about preserving and transmitting indigenous medical knowledge, and they insist that they are prepared to collaborate with those who would want to carry out action-oriented research and explore opportunities for co-operation.

For this to happen, however, they argue that it is essential first to establish genuine healers associations organised by healers that can certify qualified practitioners, promote members' interests, and create harmonious working relationships with the Ministry of Health and other governmental bodies. While healers associations were created in the past, they were largely ineffectual and dominated by the state. They thus generated little enthusiasm.

In addition to building strong healers association, creating a favourable working environment for healers free from state harassment, is an extremely important precondition for learned healers to come forward and participate in developing an integrated health system.

Many cleric–healers also recognise that they need to provide evidence of the hypothetical association between the material and non-material elements of their therapies and their pragmatic worth. In addition, they acknowledge that any effort to develop an integrated system of medical care will require healers to work together to systematise church-based medical knowledge. The evolution of multiple forms of medical care loosely based on church-based medicine over the course of the twentieth century has created a situation in which it is unclear just what ideas and practices constitute church-based healing, and thus what should be integrated into the healthcare system. Among the work that needs to be done in this regard is the adoption of linguistic standards for the supposedly unintelligible words and phrases, and the mysterious writing technique called *nagara dabtara.* This collaborative effort would also aim to produce new standardised magico-medical texts; in other words, caring for the literate healing tradition is the same as caring for the healthcare needs of the majority of the population. It is only with cleric healers' wholehearted participation and scrupulous examination of magico-medical texts that the flaws and deficiencies of the written knowledge that have occurred over the twentieth century can be redressed. By the same token, such an endeavour would help researchers to appreciate the peculiarity of the Ethiopian church-based therapeutic modalities vis-à-vis the various schools of healing traditions that had been functioning and documented in different parts of the world.

At the moment, however, such a collaborative effort is far from becoming a reality. Many healers remain resistant to departing from a tradition in which medical knowledge and its transmission have been closeted in secrecy. Moreover, many of those who possess knowledge of church-based medicine are growing old and there may not be time to develop the type of long-term collaborative project proposed here.

Even the first step of creating healers associations that would begin the necessary collaborative work faces many challenges.

All previous attempts at setting up healers associations have been partially obstructed by practitioners' deep-rooted suspicion of one another, their lack of faith in the intentions of the state and, above all, their lack of freedom to organise autonomous healers associations with legitimate and trusted leadership. Informants admitted that during the imperial era most cleric–healers were extremely egoistical and more interested in outsmarting their competitors than doing something to promote their collective rights and interests.[1]

Later, the unpleasant experience of the Darg period deprived cleric–healers of their sense of community at the same time as it alienated them from any government involvement or initiative in matters relating to indigenous medicine and healing. The military government stigmatised *dabtara* cleric–healers and prevented them from taking part in its Primary Healthcare Programme. At the same time, cleric–healers viewed the Darg as contributing to the burgeoning of non-cleric–healers as well as 'self-styled' cleric–healers (*margeta*). During this time, any person claiming to be a healer was free to acquire an identification or registration paper from one of the supposedly independent healers associations. To obtain registration papers, it would suffice for an applicant to have a letter verifying his permanent address from his local urban or farmers' association.

For cleric–healers, the absence of legitimate healer associations meant that there was no mechanism for regulating the qualifications of cleric or non-cleric–healers. The state organised associations established under the Darg were viewed as incompetent and unable to regulate the field. They were seen instead as assisting scores of inept healers to acquire identification or registration papers and work permits, and flood the urban medical marketplace. This corrupted the practice of church-based medicine while challenging the position of legitimate cleric–healers in the medical marketplace.

Cleric–healer mistrust and scepticism of government initiatives in traditional medicine created during the Darg period have continued into the post-Darg years. At the same time, post-Darg governments have not significantly altered Darg policies regarding the treatment of indigenous healers. The post-1991 regime, parading itself as a promoter of a new policy based on cultural, religious, linguistic and regional differences of the country's multi-ethnic population, has done little to promote the strong culturally based system of medical knowledge that is the basis of church-based healing. At the same time, the policy of regionalism has stood in the way of the development of a national healers association.

Thus, despite the public's faith and confidence in indigenous healing practices, many cleric–healers are troubled by the continued underutilisation of church-based medico-magical knowledge, and by the gradual loss of qualified healers, as knowledgeable healers pass away and fewer and fewer new healers are being trained. More importantly, cleric–healers are most concerned about the damage inflicted on the reputation of church-based healing by individuals who wish to discredit church-based healers by emphasising the harmful and unethical actions of the many fraudulent, ill-trained practitioners who claim to be practising church-based medicine.

The barriers to developing an effective integration of indigenous healing traditions and primary health care in Ethiopia have deep roots stretching back to the early introduction of Western medicine and education under Menelik II. Any effort to overcome the obstacles to integration need to understand this longer history and how it has transformed indigenous medical practices, reshaped the medical marketplace, and defined the attitudes of both church-based healers and the state.

Notes

1 Wondwosen Teshome-Bahiru, 'Impacts of Urbanisation on the Traditional Medicine of Ethiopia', *Anthropologist* 8(1) (2005): pp. 45–47.

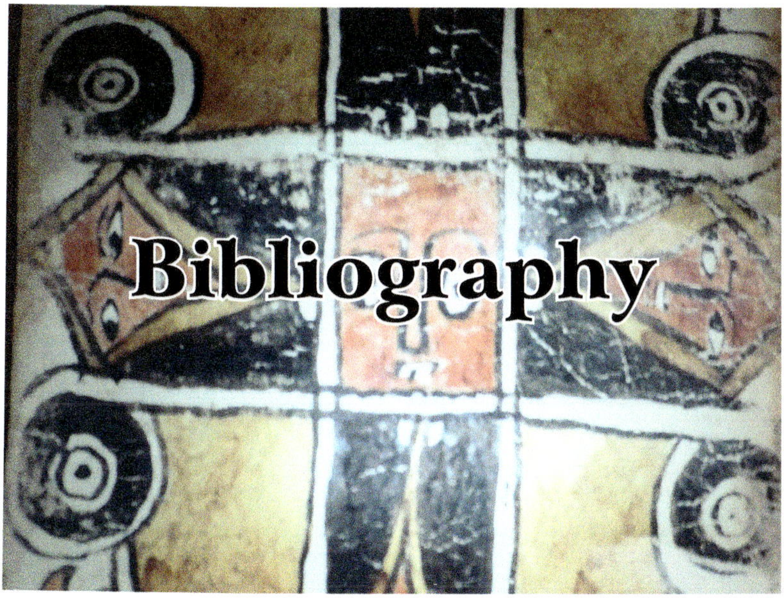

Bibliography

Abate, Gelahun. Book of Herbs: Ethiopian Traditional Medicine (Amharic). Addis Ababa: Artistic Printing Press, 1989.

Abdalla, Ismail. 'The Ulama of Sokoto in the Nineteenth Century: A Medical View'. In African Healing Strategies, edited by Brian du Toit and Ismail Abdalla, pp. 8–19. New York: Trado-Medic Books, 1985.

______. Islam, Medicine, and Practitioners in Northern Nigeria. New York, NY: The Edwin Mellen Press, 1997.

Abebe, Cherie. 'A Brief History of Mekane-Eyesus Church in South Gondar'. Unpublished B.Th. thesis. Holy Trinity Theological College, Addis Ababa, 2002.

Abebe, Dawit and Ahadu Ayehu. Medicinal Plants and Enigmatic Health Practices of Northern Ethiopia. Addis Ababa: Berhanena Salam Printing Press, 1993.

Aberra, Abayneh. Fikare Kewakebt (Occult and Mysticism) (Amharic). 2nd edition. Addis Ababa: Neged Printing Press, 1996 E.C.

Abir, Mordechai. Ethiopia and the Red Sea: The Rise and Decline of the Solomonic Dynasty and Muslim-European Rivalry in the Region. London: Frank Cass and Company Limited, 1980

Abraha, Zamanfas Qedus. Tagsatsena Mekir (Reprimand and Advice) (Amharic). 2nd edition. Asmara: Artigraphic Printing Press, 1945 E.C.

______. *Hatata Menafist za Awda Nagast.* (Amharic). 2nd edition. Asmara: El Poligraphic Association, 1948 E.C.

Abraha, Zenebe. *Manafist* (Spirits) (Amharic). Addis Ababa: Berhanena Selam Printing Press, 1992 E.C.

Adane, Tegbaru. 'A Brief History of Dima-Giyorgis Monastery'. Unpublished B.Th. thesis. Holy Trinity Theological College, Addis Ababa, 2002.

Addis Zemen, 3 September 1975; 15, 19, 20 October 1976; 6, 19, 11, 22, 23, 25 December 1976; 8 January 1977; 3,4 February 1977; 22 May 1977; 2, 3 June 1977; 25 October 1977; 26 February 1978; 13 April 1978; 29 September 1978, 2 October 1978; 29 November 1978; 3 August 1989; 17 August 1989; 24 December 1992.

Ademuwagun, Z. A, John A. A. Ayoade, Ira E. Harrison and Dennis M. Warren (eds). *African Therapeutic Systems.* Waltham, MA: Crossroads Press, 1979.

Admassu, Seyfy. 'Tesfa Gebre Selassie and His Printing Press' (Amharic). Unpublished B.A. thesis. Addis Ababa University, Addis Ababa, 1987.

Akerele, Olayiwola. 'The Best of Both Worlds: Bringing Traditional Medicine up to Date'. *Social Science and Medicine*, 24(2), 1987: pp. 177–181.

Alelegn, Mersha. *A Brief Biography of Ethiopian Bishops* (Amharic). Addis Ababa: Ethio Tikur Abbay Printers, 2005 E.C.

Almeida, Manoel de. *Some Records of Ethiopia, 1593–1646.* Revised and edited by C. F. Beckingham and G. W. B. Huntingford. London: Hakluyt Society, 1954.

Alvarez, Francisco. *The Prester John of the Indies.* 2 volumes. Revised and edited by C. F. Beckingham and G. W. B. Huntingford. Cambridge: The University Press, 1961.

Amare, Germa. 'Education and the Conflict of Values in Ethiopia: A Study of the Socio-Moral Problems Arising Out of the Introduction of Modern Education in Ethiopia'. Unpublished Ph.D. dissertation. Southern Illinois University, 1964.

Amare, Getahun, 'Some Common Medicinal and Poisonous Plants Used in Ethiopian Folk Medicine'. Mimeograph, Addis Ababa University, 1976.

Anneratone, Carlo. *Abissinia.* Rome: Enrico Voghera, 1914.

Anonymous, *The Patriots' Struggle with the Fascists* (Amharic). Addis Ababa: Berhanena Selam Printing Press, 1941 E.C.

Aseffa, Habte Mariam, *Questions on the History and Cultures of Ethiopia* (Amharic). Addis Ababa, 1986 E.C.

Asme, Giyorgis, 'Yagalla Tarik' (History of the Galla) (Amharic). Addis Ababa: IES, MS no. 173.

Aspen, Harald. *Mediums and Human Worlds: The Amhara Peasants of the North Ethiopian Highlands and Their Traditions of Knowledge.* Unpublished Ph.D. dissertation, University of Trondhein, 1994.

Awda Nagast, 1953E.C.

Ayehu, Ahadu. 'Book of Herbs' (Amharic). IES. Unpublished MS, 1990.

Bakke, Johnny. *Christian Ministry: Pattern and Functions Within the Ethiopian Evangelical Church Mekane Yesus.* Atlantic Highlands, NJ: Humanities Press International, 1987.

Bakur, 12 March 1998.

Balcha, Assefa. 'Traditional Medicine in Wallo: Its Nature and History'. Unpublished M.A. thesis. Addis Ababa University, 1992.

Bannermann, R. H., Burton, J. and W. C. Chen. *Traditional Medicine and Health Care Coverage.* Geneva: WHO, 1983.

Basset, Rene. *Les apocryphes ethiopiens.* IV *Les legends de St. Tergat et de St. Sousnyos*, 1894; V *Les prieres de la Vierge a Bartos et au Golgotha*, 1895; VI *Les Prieres de St. Cyprien et de St. Theoplile*, 1896; VII *Les apocryphes ethiopiens*, 1896. Paris: Librairie de L'Art Independent.

Bauer, Dan and John Hinnant, 'Normal and Revolutionary Divination: A Kuhnian Approach to African Systems of Thought'. In *Explorations of African Systems of Thought*, edited by Ivan Karp and Charles Bird, 213–236. Bloomington IN: Indiana University Press, 1979.

Bauer, Dan. 'The Sacred and the Secret: Order and Chaos in Tigray Medicine and Politics'. In *Creativity of Power*, edited by W. Arens and Ivan Karp. Washington: DC: Smithsonian Institution Press, 1989.

Baykedagne, Gebre Hiywot. *Emperor Menelik and Ethiopia* (Amharic). Addis Ababa: United Printers, 1993.

Berhane, Girmay. 'The *Dabtara* Doctor "*Asmat*" (Amharic). Unpublished B.A. thesis, HSIU, 1970.

Berhanu, Gebre Selassie. *Hatata Manafist WaAwda Nagast Kanatalsamu* (Amharic). Addis Ababa: Aksum Printing Press, 1997 E.C.

Berhanu, Leykun. *Tsetset* (Remorse) (Amharic). Addis Ababa: Neged Printing Press, 1999 E.C.

Beyene, Asmelash. 'Some Notes on the Evolution of Regional Administration in Ethiopia.' *Ethiopian Journal of Development Research*, 9(1), 1987: pp. 21–49.

Bishaw, Mekonnen. 'Integrating Indigenous and Cosmopolitan Medicine in Ethiopia'. Unpublished Ph.D. dissertation. Southern Illinois University, 1988.

______. 'Attitudes of Modern and Traditional Medical Practitioners toward Cooperation'. *EMJ* 28, 1990: pp. 63–72.

______. 'Promoting Traditional Medicine in Ethiopia: A Brief Historical Review of Government Policy'. *SSM* 33(2), 1991: pp. 193–200.

Brielli, D., V. Calo, A. Bevilacqua. *Note di patologia ethiopica.* Rome: Tipog. Naz. Bertero, 1912.

Brooks, Kenneth. 'Literacy in Ethiopia'. *EJE* 4(1), 1970: pp. 16–39.

Bruce, James. *Travels to Discover the Source of the Nile in the Years 1768, 1769, 1770 1771, 1772, and 1773.* 5 volumes. London: G. G. J. and J. Robinson, 1970.

Budge, Wallis. *The Book of the Saints of the Ethiopian Church*, 4 volumes. Cambridge: Cambridge University Press 1928.

______. *Bandlet of Righteousness: An Ethiopian Book of the Dead.* London: Luzac & Co., 1929.

______. *Amulets and Superstitions.* London: Humphrey Hilford, 1930.

Campbell, Ian. *The Plot to Kill Graziani: The Attempted Assassination of Mussolini's Viceroy.* Addis Ababa: Addis Ababa University Press, 2010.

Carlson, Andrew J. and Dennis G. Carlson, *Health, Wealth, and Family in Rural Ethiopia: Kossoye, North Gondar Region, 1963–2007.* Addis Ababa: Addis Ababa University Press, 2008.

Chaine, Marius. *Catalogue des Manuscrits Ethiopiens de la Collection Antoine D'Abbadie.* Paris: Imprimerie Nationale, 1912.

______. 'Catalogue des Manuscripts Ethiopiens des Bibliotheques et Musees de Paris'. *ROC*, 1914.

Chaillot, Kristin. *The Ethiopian Orthodox Tewahedo Church Tradition: A Brief Introduction to Its Life and Spirituality* (Amharic). Translated by Dagnachew Kassahun. Addis Ababa: Mahbere Qedusan, 1999 E.C.

Chang, Wen-Pin 'Development of Basic Health Services in Ethiopia'. Reprinted from the *Journal of the Formosan Medical Association* 68(6), 1969: pp. 306–321.

Chavunduka, Gordon. *Traditional Medicine in Zimbabwe.* Harare: University of Zimbabwe, 1994.

Chi, Chunhuei. 'Integrating Traditional Medicine into Modern Health Care Systems: Examining the Role of Chinese Medicine in Taiwan'. *Social Science and Medicine* 39(3), 1994: pp. 307–321.

Cohen, Marcel. 'Ceremonies et Croyances Abyssines' *Revue de l'histoire des religions*, 1912.

Conti Rossini, Carlo. 'La Redazione Etiopica della Preghiera della Vergine Fra i Parti'. *RRAL* 5, 1895: pp. 457–476.

______. 'Lo 'Awda Nagast' scritto divinatorio etiopico'. *RSE* II, 1942: pp. 127–145.

Crummey, Donald. 'The Politics of Modernization: Protestant and Catholic Missionaries in Modern Ethiopia'. In *The Missionary Factor in Ethiopia*, edited by Getachew Haile et al., pp. 85–99. Frankfurt am Main: Studien zur Interkulturellen Geschichte des Christentums, no. 119, 1998.

______. *Land and Society in the Christian Kingdom of Ethiopia: From the Thirteenth to the Twentieth Century.* Addis Ababa: Addis Ababa University Press, 2000.

D'Abbadie, Antoine. *Catalogue Raisonné de Manuscrits Ethiopiens.* Paris, 1859.

Dagne, Haile Gabriel. 'Education Magic in Traditional Ethiopia'. *EJE* 4(2), 1971: pp. 3–12.

Debebe, Wossen. *Tesfa Gebre Selassie of Bulga* (Amharic). Addis Ababa: Tesfa Gebre Selassie Printing Press, 2004 EC.

De Castro, Lincoln. *Nella Terra Dei Negus.* Milan: Fratelli Treves, 1915.

Deribe, Kebede et al. 'A Historical Overview of Traditional Medicine Practices and Policy in Ethiopia'. *Ethiopian Journal of Health Development*, 20(2), 2006: pp. 127–134.

Dillmann, August. *Catalogus Codicum Manuscriptorum Orientalium qui in Museo Britannico asservantur.* Pars tertia. London, 1847.

_______. *Catalogus Codicum Manuscriptorum Bibliothecae Oxoniensis.* Pars vii, 1848.

_______. *Ethiopic Grammar.* Translated by A. Crichton. London: Williams & Norgate, 1907.

Doresse, Jean. *Ethiopia: Ancient Cities and Temples.* London: Elek Books, 1959.

Eide, Oyvind. *Revolution and Religion in Ethiopia.* Oxford: James Currey, 2000.

Enchalew, Merawi. 'A Brief History of Mahbere Selassie Monastery'. Unpublished B.Th. thesis. Holy Trinity Theological College, Addis Ababa, 2000.

Endeshaw, Assafa. *Ethiopia: Perspectives for Change and Renewal.* Singapore: Seng Lee Press, 2002.

Engdasew, Agonafer. A speech delivered at the 7th Regular Conference of the Ethiopian Medical Association, Addis Ababa, Unpublished MS, n.d.

______. A speech delivered at the August Conference of the Ethiopian Health and Nutrition Research Institute, Addis Ababa, Unpublished MS, n.d.

Engeda, Fantahun. *Major Political Problems and Struggles During Haile Selassie's Administration as Learned from the Biography of the Emperor's Close Associates* (Amharic). Addis Ababa: Berhanena Selam Printing Press, 1997 E.C.

Ermias Kebede (Nebura ed.). *Ethiopia and Ethiopianness* (Amharic). Addis Ababa: Chamber Printing Press, 2004.

Euringer, Sebastien. 'Une priere pour conjurer les demons'. *ROC*, XXIII, 1922–1923.

______. 'L'hymne-invocation lessane sab'e'. *Aethiopica*, 1935.

______. 'La priere Sayfa Malakot'. *Aethiopica*, 1936.

______. 'Die Binde der Rechtfertigung (Lefafa Tsedek)'. *Orientali*, IX, 1940.

Feierman, Steven. 'The Social Origins of Health and Healing in Africa'. Paper Presented at the 27th Annual Meeting of the African Studies Association, 25–28 October 1984, Los Angeles, CA.

______. *Peasant Intellectuals: Anthropology and History in Tanzania.* Madison: The University of Wisconsin Press, 1990.

Feierman, Steven and John Janzen (eds). *The Social Basis of Health and Healing in Africa.* Berkeley: University of California Press, 1992.

Flint, Karen. 'Competition, Race, and Professionalization: African Healers and White Medical Practitioners in Natal, South Africa in the Early Twentieth Century'. The *Society for the Social History of Medicine* 14(2), 2001: pp. 199–221.

______. 'Indian-African Encounters: Polyculturalism and African Therapeutics in Natal, South Africa, 1886–1950s'. *Journal of South African Studies* 32(2), 2006: pp. 367–385.

F.O. 371, no. 41498, A Report by A. F. Mathew, October 1943.

Fries, Karl. 'The Ethiopic Legend of Socinius und Ursule'. *Actes du VIIIe Congres International des Orientalistes.* Section I B, Leiden, 1893.

Fullas, Fekadu. 'The Role of Indigenous Medicinal Plants in Ethiopian Healthcare'. *African Renaissance*, 2007.

Gadlie, Taddele. *Qene and Qene Games to Cherish the Past.* 2nd edition. (Amharic). Addis Ababa: Gutenberg Printing Press, 1997 E.C.

Gebre, Temesgen. *Autobiography* (Amharic). Addis Ababa: Alpha Printers, 2001 E.C.

Gebre Ab, Tesfaye. *Qoritoch at Bishaftu* (Amharic). Addis Ababa: Commercial Printing Press, 2001.

Gebre Mariam, Gebre Yohannes. *Taqwame Mahtot* (literally 'Candle Burner') (Amharic). Addis Ababa: Tensae Zegubae Printing Press, 1992 E.C.

Gebre Meskel, Haddis (ed.). *Book of Medicine: Traditional Ethiopian Medicine* (Amharic). London: Haddis Publications, 1988.

Geest, Sjaak van der. 'Is There a Role for Traditional Medicine in Basic Health Service in Africa? A Plea for a Community Perspective'. *Tropical Medicine and International Health* 2(9), 1997: pp. 903–911.

Gelfand, Michael. *Witch Doctor: Traditional Medicine Man of Rhodesia.* New York: Frederick A. Praeger, 1965.

Getachew, Gezahegn. 'The Various Characters of the Hagiographies' (Amharic). In *Proceedings of the Workshop on the Ethiopian Church Yesterday, Today and Tomorrow*, Addis Ababa, 18–19 April 2002.

Getahun, Kidane Mariam. *The Traditional Religious Student* (Amharic). Addis Ababa: Tensae Zagubae Printing Press, 1954 E.C.

Giday, Yitbarek. *My Life and the Qene Bet Tradition* (Amharic). Addis Ababa: Artistic Printing Press, n.d.

Gobat, Samuel. *Journal of the Three Years' Residence in Abyssinia.* London: Hatchard & Son Seeley & Sons, 1834.

Good, C. M. *Ethnomedical Systems in Africa: Patterns of Traditional Medicine in Rural and Urban Kenya.* New York: Guilford Press, 1978.

Goody, Jack. *The Interface Between the Written and the Oral.* Cambridge: Cambridge University Press, 1987.

Grebaut, Sylvain. 'Noms ésotériques de Dieu rêvéles aux archanges'. *Aethiopica*, 1934.

______. 'Priere magique contre la dysenterie'. *Aethiopica*, 1934.

______. 'L' hymne: Invocation Lesana Sab'e. *Aethiopica*, 1935.

______. 'Le prière Sayfa Malakot'. *Aethiopica*, 1936.

______. 'Priere contre la pleuresie'. *Aethiopica*, 1936.

______. 'Priere magique contre le feu'. *Aethiopica*, 1936.

______. 'Priere magique contre la grele'. *Aethiopica*, 1938.

______. *Recueil de texts magique ethiopiens.* Paris: Librairie Orientaliste Paul Geuthner, 1939.

Grebaut, Sylvain and Evgenivs Tisserant, *Codices Aethiopici Vaticani et Borgiani.* Vatican, 1935.

Green, Edward and Lydia Makhubu, 'Traditional Healers in Swaziland: Toward Improved Cooperation between the Traditional and Modern Health Sectors'. *Social Science and Medicine* 18(12), 1984: pp. 1071–1079.

Greenfield, Richard. *Ethiopia: A New Political History.* London: Pall Mall Press, 1965.

Griaule, Marcel. 'Mythes, croyances et coutumes de Begameder (Abyssinie)'. *Journal Asiatique*, 1928: 19–124.

______. *Le livre de recettes d'un dabtara abyssin.* Paris: Institut d'Ethnologie, 1930.

______. 'Le travail en Abyssinie'. *Revue Internationale du Travai* 23(2), 1931.

______. 'Les règles de l'eglise'. *Journal Asiatique* 221, 1932: pp. 31–33.

______. 'Notes sur l'arithmomancie ethiopiennne'. *Journal de la Societe des Africanistes* IV, 1934: pp. 25–31.

Haile Selassie Foundation. *Haile Selassie I Foundation: 1945–1965* (Amharic). Addis Ababa: Berhanena Selam Printing Press, 1965 E.C.

Haile Selassie, Imru. *From What I Heard and Remember* (Amharic). Addis Ababa: Addis Ababa University Press, 2001, E.C.

Haile, Getachew (ed.) *The Works of Abba Bahriy with Other Documents Concerning the Oromo* (Amharic and English). Addis Ababa, 2005.

Hamar, November/December 1994 E.C.; May/June 1994 E.C.; May/June 1995 E.C.

Handloff, Robert. 'Prayers, Amulets, and Charms: Health and Social Control'. *The African Studies Review* 25, 1982: 185–194.

Harris, Cornwallis. *The Highlands of Ethiopia*, II. 2nd edition. London: Longman, Brown, Green and Longman, 1844.

Hayes, Arthur. *The Source of the Blue Nile*. London: Smith, Elder & Co., 1905.

Hedaru, Hiywot. *Those Days Have Been Forgotten: From School to Consular Work 1932–1941* (Amharic). Addis Ababa: Berhanena Selam Printing Press, 1967 E.C.

Henze, Paul. 'Movement Toward Modernization: A Century of Progress'. In *The Ecology of Health and Disease in Ethiopia*, edited by Helmut Kloos and Zein Ahmed Zein, pp. 79–103. Colorado: Westview Press, 1993.

Hotten, John (ed.). *Abyssinia and Its People*. New York: Negro University Press, 1969.

IEG *see* Imperial Ethiopian Government.

IES *see* Institute of Ethiopian Studies.

Imperato, Pascal James. *African Folk Medicine: Practices and Beliefs of the Bambara and Other People*. Baltimore: York Press, 1977.

Imperial Ethiopian Government. *Nagarit Gazeta*, Proclamation no. 27. October 1942.

_______. *Nagarit Gazeta*, 'Regulation for the Administration of the Church'. November 1942.

_______. *Nagarit Gazeta*, Decree no. 1 of 1942.

_______. *Negarit Gazeta*, Proclamation no. 1. September 1948.

_______. *Negarit Gazeta*, *Penal Code of 1957*.

_______. *Negarit Gazeta*, Order no. 22 of 1960.

Institute of Ethiopian Studies, Addis Ababa University. MSS nos. 79, 127, 141, 144–148, 151, 155–159, 162–172, 178–179, 181,

186, 190–192, 195, 210, 217–221, 224–239, 244, 296, 330, 345, 386, 403–416, 437, 445–456, 458–459, 463, 473–492, 495, 498, 500–674, 680, 698, 785, 792, 795, 992, 1020, 1053, 1056, 1065, 1067, 1068, 1082, 1782, 1990, 1998, 2151, 2153, 2183–2184, 2193, 2199, 2204, 2210, 2213, 2243, 2244, 2262, 2310, 2378, 2417 (A, B, C, D, E, F, H, I, J, Ka, Kb, La, Lb, N, O&P), 2444, 2481, 2595, 2694, 2695, 2938–2939, 2976, 3000–3002, 3007, 3983.

Janzen, John. *The Quest for Therapy in Lower Zaire*. Berkeley: University of California, 1978.

______. *Lemba, 1650–1030: A Drum of Affliction in Africa and the New World*. New York: Garland Publishing, 1982.

______. *Ngoma: Discourses of Healing in Central and Southern Africa*. Berkeley: University of California Press, 1992.

Jembere, Admassu. *Kokeha Haimanot* (Strong Religion) (Amharic). Addis Ababa: Tensae Zagubae Printing Press, 1949 E.C.

Jemberre, Abera. *Establishment of the Haile Selassie I Foundation* (Amharic). Addis Ababa: Berhanena Selam Printing Press, 1952 E.C.

Johnston, Charles. *Travels in Southern Abyssini*. Volume II. London: J. Madden & Co., 1844.

Kallacha, Walda Mikael. *A Glossary of Ethiopian Plant Names*. 4th edition. Addis Ababa: Artistic Printers, 1987.

Kassaw, Bitew. 'Migration of Clergymen from Rural Areas to the Cities: The Case in Addis'. Unpublished B.Th. thesis. Holy Trinity Theological College, Addis Ababa, 2001.

Katz, Sydney, Selig Katz and Violet Kimani. 'The Making of an Urban Mganga: New Trends in Traditional Medicine in Urban Kenya'. *Medical Anthropology* 6(2), 1982: pp. 91–112.

Kebebew, Fassil. 'The Status and Availability of Data of Oral and Written Knowledge on Traditional Health Care in Ethiopia'. In *Proceedings of the National Workshop on Conservation and Sustainable Use of Medicinal Plants in Ethiopia*, Addis Ababa, 28 April–May 1998.

Kebede, Berihun. *History of Emperor Haile Selassie* (Amharic). Addis Ababa: Artistic Printing Press, 1993 E.C.

Kebede, Genet. Church Schools (Amharic). In *Proceedings of the Workshop on the Ethiopian Church Yesterday, Today and Tomorrow*, Addis Ababa, 18–19 April 2002.

Kebede, Mesele Terecha. *Leprosy, Leprosaria and Society in Ethiopia*. Addis Ababa: The Armaeur Hansen Research Institute, 2008.

Kefyalew, Dawit. 'Spirit and Spirits: Inspiration of the Holies'. Unpublished B.Th. thesis. Holy Trinity Theological College, Addis Ababa, 1999.

Kibret, Daniel (ed.), *Church Documents* (Amharic). Volume I. Addis Ababa: Mega Printing Enterprise, 1999 E.C.

Kieckhefer, Richard, *Magic in the Middle Ages*. Cambridge: Cambridge University Press, 1989, p. 89.

Kifle, Kidane Wold. *Book of Grammar and the New Ge'ez Etymological Dictionary* (Amharic). Addis Ababa: Artistic Printing Press, 1948 E.C.

Kimani, V. N. 'The Unsystematic Alternative: Towards Plural Health Care among the Kikuyu of Central Kenya'. *SSM*. 15B, 1981.

Kirk, R. 'Medical Report on the Kingdom of Shoa'. *Transactions of the Medical and Physical Society of Bombay*, 1843.

Kloos, Helmut and Zein Ahmed Zein (eds.). *The Ecology of Health and Disease in Ethiopia*. Colorado: Westview Press, 1993.

Kloos, Helmut et al. 'The Geography of Pharmacies, Druggist Shops, and Rural Medicine Vendors, and the Origin of Customers to such Facilities in Addis Ababa'. *JES* 12(2), 1974: pp. 77–94.

Lalalet, Yewelsew. 'The *Awaqi* and His Magical Activities around the Dabra Marqos Area' (Amharic). Unpublished B.A. thesis. Addis Ababa University, Addis Ababa, 1992.

Lamin, Sanneh. *The Jakhanke: The History of an Islamic Clerical People of the Senegambia*. London: International African Institute, 1979.

Leiris, M. 'La croyance aux genies 'Zar' en Ethiopie du Nord'. n.p.

______. 'Le culte des Zars a Gondar'. *Aethiopica*, 1934

______. 'Un rite medico-magique ethiopien: Le jet de Danqara'. *Aethiopica*, 1934.

Lemordant, D. *Les plantes Ethiopiennes*. Addis Ababa: Central Printing Press, 1960.

Levine, Donald. *Wax and Gold: Tradition and Innovation in Ethiopian Culture*. Chicago: The University of Chicago Press, 1965.

______. *Greater Ethiopia: The Evolution of a Multiethnic Society*. Chicago: The University of Chicago Press, 1974.

Lewis, I. M. *Religion in Context*. Cambridge, Cambridge University Press, 1986.

Libsework, Tekle. 'A Brief History of Bethlehem Church (South Gondar)'. Unpublished B.Th. thesis. Holy Trinity Theological College, Addis Ababa, 2002.

Lifchitz, Deborah. *Textes ethioipiens magico-religieux*. Paris: Institut d'Ethnologie, 1940.

Littmann, Enno. 'The Princeton Ethiopic Magic Scroll'. *Princeton University Bulletin*, XV, 1, December 1903.

______. 'Arde'et: The Magic Book of the Disciples'. *JAOS*. XXV, 1904.

Ludolph, Joab. *The New History of Ethiopia*. 2nd edition. London: S. Smith, 1684.

Makinde, Akin. *African Philosophy, Culture, and Traditional Medicine*. Athens: Ohio University, 1988.

Mariam, Taye Gebre (Alaqa). *History of the People of Ethiopia* (Amharic). 6th edition. Addis Ababa: Qedus Giyorgis Printing Press, 1958 E.C.

Markakis, John. *Ethiopia: Anatomy of a Traditional Polity*. Oxford: Clarendon Press, 1974.

Mateqe, June, 2005.

Mekonnen, Girma. 'Literacy and Libraries in Ethiopia'. Unpublished M.A. thesis. Loughborough University of Technology, 1983.

Mekuria, Tekle Tsadik. *Human Behavior and Techniques on Social Life* (Amharic). Addis Ababa: Tensae Zagubae Printing Press, 1951.

______. *History of Ethiopia: From Emperor Lebne Dengel to Emperor Tewodros* (Amharic). Addis Ababa: Tensae Zagubae Printing Press, 1953 E.C.

______. *The Wars of Ahmed Gragne* (Amharic). Addis Ababa: Berhanena Selam Printing Press, 1966 E.C.

______. *Emperor Menelik and Ethiopia's Unity* (Amharic). Addis Ababa: Kuraz Publishing Agency, 1983 E.C.

Mengistu, Girma. 'The Poems of Alaqa Inbaqom Kalawold' (Amharic). Unpublished B.A. thesis. Addis Ababa University, Addis Ababa, 1987.

Mérab, Paul. *Medecins et medecine en Ethiopie.* Paris: Vigot Fréres, 1912.

______. *Impressions d'Ethiopie 1921–1929.* Volume III. Paris: Editions Ernest Leroux, 1921–1929.

Mercier, Jacques. 'Les Däbtära et le vocabulaire de la magie et de la medecine'. *Documents Histoire Civilisation Ethiopienne, RCP* 230, 1976.

______. *Ethiopian Magic Scrolls.* New York: George Braziller Inc., 1979.

______. 'Les hallucinogenes ethiopiens identification'. *Abbay.* 10, 1979.

______. *Rouleaux magiques ethiopiens.* Paris: Editions du Seuil, 1979.

______. 'Le Traité medical de Gelahun Abate'. *Abbay.* 12, 1983–84.

______. *Asres: Le magicien ethiopien.* Paris: Jean-Claude Lattes, 1988.

______. *Art That Heals: The Image as Medicine in Ethiopia.* New York: The Museum of African Art, 1997.

Messing, Simon. 'The Highland Plateau Amhara of Ethiopia'. Unpublished Ph.D. dissertation. University of Pennsylvania, 1957.

Ministry of Education, *Physiology and Hygiene* (Amharic). Volume 1. Addis Ababa: Berhanena Selam Printing Press, 1934 E.C.

Ministry of Health. Health Policy of the Transitional Government of Ethiopia, September 1993.

______. National Drug Policy of the Transitional Government of Ethiopia, November 1993.

Ministry of Interior, file no. 4/2, G. G. Campbell, Director-General of Medical Services, 'Memorandum for the U.N.R.R.A. Mission to Ethiopia'. 11 February 1946.

Ministry of Public Health. 'Directory of Medical and Health Institutions in Ethiopia'. Addis Ababa, January, 1972.

______. *Health Facilities and Personnel in Ethiopia.* Addis Ababa, September, 1972.

______. *Proceedings of the First National Conference on Ethiopian Traditional Medicine and Healing* (Amharic). Addis Ababa, 27–29 June 1980.

Moges, Alemayehu. 'The Traditional Church Education'. Unpublished B.Th. thesis. Holy Trinity Theological College, Addis Ababa, 1971.

______. 'Traditional Ethiopian Medicine'. 8th International Conference of Ethiopian Studies. Volume I. Addis Ababa, 1984.

Molvaer, Reidulf. 'Medical Anthropology Topics of Relevance for Health Workers and Students of Health in Ethiopia'. Addis Ababa: UNICEF/Ministry of Health, 1987.

Mooney, N. F. *A Glossary of Ethiopian Plant Names.* Dublin: Dublin University Press, 1963.

Muluneh, Kumlachew. 'The History of Komma Fasiladas'. Unpublished B.Th. thesis. Holy Trinity Theological College, Addis Ababa, 2002.

National Archive and Library, Addis Ababa, MS no. 492.

Natvig, Richard. 'Oromos, Slaves, and the Zar Spirits: A Contribution to the History of the Zar Cult'. *The International Journal of African Historical Studies* 20(4), 1987: pp. 669–689.

Negussie, Zelalem. 'A Brief History of Zuramba Aregawi Monastery'. Unpublished B.Th. thesis. Holy Trinity Theological College, Addis Ababa, 2002.

Neumann, A. and P. Lauro. 'Ethnomedicine and Biomedicine Linking'. *Social Science and Medicine*, 16, 1982: pp. 1817–1824.

Nogngno, Pawlos. *Emperor Menelik* (Amharic). Addis Ababa: Bole Printing Press, 1984 E.C.

O'Hanlon, Douglas. *Features of the Abyssinian Church.* London: Society for Promoting Christian Knowledge, 1946.

O'Kelly, Sebastian. *Amedeo: The True Story of An Italian's War in Abyssinia*, London: Harper Collins Publishers, 2003.

Offiong, Daniel. 'Traditional Healers in the Nigerian Health Care Delivery System and the Debate over Integrating Traditional and Scientific'. *Anthropological Quarterly* 72(3), 1999: pp. 118–130.

Owusu-Ansah, David. *Islamic Talismanic Tradition in Nineteenth-Century Asante.* New York: The Edwin Mellen Press, 1991.

______. 'Prayers, Amulets, and Healing'. In *The History of Islam in Africa*, edited by Nehema Levtzion and Randall Pouwels, pp. 477–488. Athens, OH: Ohio University Press, 2000.

Packard, Randall. *The Making of a Tropical Disease: A Short History of Malaria.* Baltimore, MD: Johns Hopkins University Press, 2007.

Pankhurst, Helen. 'What Change and for Whom? The Case of Women in Menz'. In *Ethiopia: Rural Development Options*, edited by Siegfried Pausewang et al. London & New Jersey: Zed Books Ltd., 1990.

Pankhurst, Richard. *An Introduction to the Economic History of Ethiopia from Early Times to 1800*. London; Lalibela House, 1961.

______ . 'The Foundations of Education, Printing, Newspaper, Book Production, Libraries and Literacy in Ethiopia'. *Ethiopian Observer* 6(3), 1962: 241–292.

______. 'The History and Traditional Treatment of Small-pox in Ethiopia'. *Medical History* 9(4), 1965: pp. 343–355.

______. 'The Beginnings of Modern Medicine in Ethiopia'. *Ethiopian Observer* 9(2), 1965; pp. 114–158.

______. 'Traditional Ethiopian Medicine and Surgery'. *Ethiopian Medical Journal* 3, 1965: pp. 151–172.

______. 'The Medical History of Ethiopia During the Italian Invasion and Occupation (1935–1941)'. *JES* 4(2), 1973: pp. 108–117.

______, 'Some Notes for the History of Typhus'. Mimeograph, 1975.

______. 'Historical Examination on the Traditional Ethiopian Pharmacopoeia'. Paper Presented at the Conference of the Ethiopian Pharmaceutical Association. Addis Ababa, 1975.

______. 'Old-time Ethiopian Cures for Syphilis'. Journal *of the History of Medicine and Allied Sciences* 30(3), 1975: pp. 199–216.

______. 'The Hedar Bašeta of 1918'. *JES* 13(2), 1975: pp. 103–131.

______. *A Social History of Ethiopia*. Addis Ababa: Institute of Ethiopian Studies, 1990.

______. *An Introduction to the Medical History of Ethiopia*. Trenton, NJ: The Red Sea Press, 1990.

______. 'Italian Fascist War Crimes in Ethiopia: History of Their Discussion, from the League of Nations to the United Nations (1936 1949)'. *Northeast African Studies*, 6(1–2), 1999: pp. 83–140.

Pankhurst, Sylvia. *Ethiopia: A Cultural History*. Essex: Lalibela House, 1955.

Parkyns, Mansfeld. *Life in Abyssinia*. Volume I. New York: D'Appleton & Co., 1854.

Pearce, Nathaniel. *The Life and Adventures of Nathaniel Pearce*. London: Sesor Publisher, 1831.

Perham, Margery. *The Government of Ethiopia.* London: Faber and Faber, 1947.

Pigg, Stacy. 'Acronyms and Effacement: Traditional Medical Practitioners (TMP) In International Health Development'. *Social Science and Medicine'* 41, 1995: pp. 47–68.

Pillsbury, Barbara. 'Policy and Evaluation Perspectives on Traditional Health Practitioners in National Health Care Systems'. *Social Science and Medicine* 16, 1982: pp. 1825–1834.

Plowden, Walter. *Travels in Abyssinia and the Galla Country with Account of a Mission to Ras Ali in 1848.* London: Longmans Green & Co., 1868.

Prouty, Chris. *The Medical History of Menelik II, Emperor of Ethiopia (1844–1913): A Case of Medical Diplomacy.* Pasadena, pp. 1844–1913: California Institute of Technology, 1978.

Prouty, Chris and Eugene Rosenfeld. *Historical Dictionary of Ethiopia.* Metuchen & London: The Scarecrow Press, 1981.

Qalawold, Inbaqom. 'Qene Education and its Uses' (Amharic). *Proceeding of the Third International Conference on Ethiopian Studies.* Volume 2, Addis Ababa, 1966.

Rahmato, Dessalegn. 'Environmentalism and Conservation in Wallo before the Revolution'. *JES* 31(1), 1998: pp. 43–86.

Reporter, 13 October 2003.

Retta, Zewde. *Tafari Mekonnen: His Long Journey to Power, 1892–1930* (Amharic). Addis Ababa: Central Printing Press, 1998 E.C.

Reynolds, Pamela. 'The Training of Traditional Healers in Mashonaland'. In *The Professionalisation of African Medicine*, edited by M. Last and G. L. Chavunduka, 165 187. Manchester: Manchester University Press, 1986.

Rodinson, Maxim. *Magie, medicine possession en Ethiopie.* Paris: Mouton & Co., 1967.

Rosenberg, Charles. 'Alternative to What? Complementary to Whom?' Paper Presented at the Program in the History of Science, Medicine and Technology, Johns Hopkins University, Baltimore, MD., 14 September 2006.

Ruphael, Leul Wolde, 'Herbal Medicine'. Mimeograph (Amharic), Addis Ababa: National Archives and Libraries, MS no. 492, 1983.

Sabure, Ahadu. *The Downfall of Haile Selassie I and the Rise of the Darg* (Amharic). Addis Ababa: n.p., n.d.

Sbacchi, Alberto. *Ethiopia Under Mussolini: Fascism and the Colonial Experience.* London: Zed Books, 1985.

________, *Legacy of Bitterness: Ethiopia and Fascist Italy, 1935–1941.* New Jersey, NJ: The Red Sea Press, 1997.

Selassie, Gebre (*Tsehafi Tezaz*). *A History of the Period of Menelik II, Emperor of Ethiopia* (Amharic). Addis Ababa: Artistic Printing Press, 1959 E.C.

Selassie, Haile. *My Life and Ethiopia's Progress* (Amharic). Volume 1. Bath, 1929 E.C.

Selassie, Haile. *My Life and Ethiopia's Progress* (Amharic). Volume 2. Addis Ababa: Berhanena Selam Printing Press, 1966.

Selassie, Sahle Mikael Wolde. *Traditional Medicine by Indigenous Scholars* (Amharic). Addis Ababa: Tensae Zagubae Printing Press, 1956 E.C.

Selassie, Sergew Hable (ed.), 'Amharic Church Dictionary'. Unpublished MS, IES, n.d.

Selassie, Tesfa Gebre. Publisher of the various magico-religious prayers cited in the book.

Selassie, Tilahun Berhane. *Twentieth Century Ethiopia* (Amharic). Volume 1. Addis Ababa: Artistic Printing Press, 1998 E.C.

Selassie, Tsehai Berhane. 'An Ethiopian Medical Text-book Written by Gerazmac Gabrawald Aragahan Daga Damot'. *JES* 3(1), 1971: 95–180.

Sewasw, Mistre. 'The Traditional Educational System of the Qene Schools' (Amharic). Unpublished B.A. thesis. Addis Ababa University, Addis Ababa, 1982.

Shorter, Frank. *The Conquest of Malaria, Italy, 1900–1962.* New Haven: Yale University Press, 2006.

Simon, J. 'Bibliography on Malkee'. *Orientalia* 10, 1941: pp. 285–311.

Slikkerveer, L. J. 'Rural Health Development in Ethiopia: Problems of Utilization of Traditional Healers'. *SSM* 16, 1982: pp. 1859 1872.

Stitz, V. 'Distribution and Foundation of Churches in Ethiopia'. *JES* 13(1), 1975: pp. 11–36.

Stone, Linda. 'Primary Health Care for Whom? Village Perspectives from Nepal'. *Social Science and Medicine* 22, 1986: pp. 293–302.

Strelcyn, Stefan. 'Ethiopian Medical Treatises as a Source for the Study of Early Amharic'. Translated from the French text by C. C. Patterson and A. K. Irvine, *International Congress of Africanists*, n.d.

______. *Catalogue des manuscrits ethiopiens (collection griaule)*. Tome IV. Paris: Imprimerie Nationale, 1954.

______. *Priéres magiques éthiopiennes pour dêlier les charmes (Mefthe Seray)*. Warsaw: Rocznik Orientalistyczny, 1955.

______. 'Mission scientifiqùe en Ethiopie'. *Accademia Polacca di Scienze e Lettere*. Roma, 1959.

______. 'La magie ethiopienne'. Acadamia Nazionale dei Lincei, 1960.

______. 'Les ecrits medicaux Ethiopiens'. *JES* 3(1), 1965: pp. 88–97.

______. 'Les medecines du Begamder et du Tchelga (Ethiopie) D'Abbaba Garred'. *Africana Bulletin* 5, 1966: 53–78.

______. *Medicins et plantes d'Ethiopie: Les traites medicaux ethiopiens*. Volume 1. Warazawa: Panstwowe, 1968.

______. 'Les chapitres concernant les plantes d'un lexique Arabe-Ethiopien du XVI. s'*Roczn. Orient* XXXI, 1968: pp. 7–28.

______. 'Catalogue of Ethiopian Manuscripts of the Wellcome Institute of the History of Medicine in London'. *BSOAS*, 35(1), 1972: pp. 27–55.

______. 'Les nouveaux manuscrits ethiopiens de la Bibliothèque Royale de Bruxelles'. *JES* 11(2), 1973: pp. 169–188.

______. *Medecine et plantes d'Ethiopie*. Volume 2. Naples: Instituto Universario Orientale, 1973.

______. *Catalogue of Ethiopian Manuscripts in the British Library Acquired Since the Year 1877*. London: British Museum Publications Ltd., 1978

Swartut, Hubert. *Yatena Mogzit* (Guardian of Health) (Amharic). Translated by Abebe Bezuneh. Addis Ababa: Adventist Printing Press, 1966.

Talbot, David. *Haile Selassie I: Silver Jubilee*. Hague: W. P. Van Stockum & Zoon, 1955.

Tamirat, Solomon. 'King Zara Yaeqob Defender and Protector of the Ethiopian Orthodox Tewahdo Church'.Unpublished B.Th. thesis. Holy Trinity Theological College, Addis Ababa, 1999.

Tamrat, Tadesse. *Church and State in Ethiopia 1270–1527*. Oxford: The Clarendon Press, 1972.

Tekle Wold, Desta. *New Amharic Dictionary* (Amharic). Addis Ababa: Artistic Printing Press, 1962 E.C.

Teshager Wube, 'The Wandering Student'. *Ethnography Society Bulletin* 9, 1959: pp. 52–60.

Teshome-Bahiru, Wondwosen, 'Impacts of Urbanisation on the Traditional Medicine of Ethiopia'. *Anthropologist*, 8(1), 2005: pp. 43–52.

Tesemma, Azene Bekele, A. Barnie and B. Tengnas, *Useful Trees and Shrubs for Ethiopia: Identification, Propagation and Management for Agricultural and Pastoral Communities.* Nairobi: Swedish International Development Authority, 1993.

The Ethiopian Orthodox Church. *Fetha Nagast* (Law of Kings) (Amharic).1st edition. Addis Ababa: Berhanena Selam Printing Press, 1958 E.C.

______. *Qala Awadi* (literally 'Edict Announcer') (Amharic). Addis Ababa: Tensae Zagubae Printing Press, 1971 E.C.

______. *A Short History, Faith and Order of the Ethiopian Orthodox Tewahdo Church* (Amharic). Addis Ababa: Tensae Zagubae Printing Press, 1975 E.C.

______. *Haymanote Abew* (Religion of the Fathers) (Amharic). Addis Ababa: Tensae Zagubae Printing Press, 1986 E.C.

______. *Ethiopia: for the World to Judge* (Amharic). Addis Ababa: Berhanena Selam Printing Press, 1993 E.C.

______. *The Church of Ethiopia: A Panorama of History and Spiritual Life.* Addis Ababa: A Publication of the EOC, 1997.

The Holy Bible (DC RO13) (Amharic). Addis Ababa: Berhanena Selam Printing Press, 1980 E.C.

______. King James Version.

The National Healers Association Office, Addis Ababa, 'A letter of Emperor Menelik to Alaqa Gefawossen' (Amharic). Genbot 13, 1893 E.C. (20 May 1901).

The Provisional Military Administrative Council, *Negarit Gazeta*, Proclamation no. 158, 1975.

Tolla, Bekelech. *Home-Based Therapy: Indigenous Household Treatment with Organic Drugs* (Amharic). Addis Ababa: Bole Printing Enterprise, 1999 E.C.

Touraiev, Boris. 'Lefafa Sedaq'. *Pamiatniki Efiopskoi Pismiennosti.* Volume VII. St Petersburg, 1908.

Trimingham, Spencer. *Islam in East Africa.* Oxford: Clarendon Press, 1964.

______. *Islam in Ethiopia.* London: Frank Cass & Co.Ltd. 1965.

______. *The Influence of Islam Upon Africa.* London: Longman, 1968.

______. *Islam in West Africa.* Oxford: The Clarendon Press, 1972.

Tsey, Komila. 'Traditional Medicine in Contemporary Ghana: A Public Policy Analysis'. *Social Science and Medicine,* 45(7), 1997: pp. 1065–1074.

Ulin, Priscilla. 'The Traditional Healers of Botswana in Changing Society'. *Rural Africana* 26, 1974–1975: pp. 123–130.

Ullendorff, Edward. *Catalogue of Ethiopian Manuscripts in Bodleian Library.* Volume II. Oxford: The Clarendon Press, 1951.

______. *The Ethiopians: An Introduction to Country and People.* 2nd edition. London: Oxford University Press, 1965.

Ullendorff, Edward and Stephen Wright. *Catalogue of Ethiopian Manuscripts in the Cambridge University Library.* Cambridge: Cambridge University Press, 1961.

Vecchiato, Norbert. 'Traditional Medicine'. In *The Ecology of Health and Disease in Ethiopia,* edited by Helmut Kloos and Zein Ahmed Zein. Colorado: Westview Press, 1993.

Velimirovi, B. 'Is Integration of Traditional and Western Medicine Really Possible?' In *Anthropology and Primary Health Care,* edited by J. Coreil and J. D. Mull. Boulder, CO: West View Press, 1990.

Voice of Eritrea, no. 186, 30 April 1948.

Waldayes, Asrat. 'The Postliberation Period (1941–1973)'. In *An Introduction to the Medical History of Ethiopia,* edited by Richard Pankhurst, Trenton, NJ: The Red Sea Press, 1990.

Waldmeier, Theophilius. *Autobiography.* London: The Orphans Printing Press, 1925.

Walker, C.H. *The Abyssinian at Home,* London: The Sheldon Press, 1933.

Warren, Dennis. 'Bono Traditional Healers'. *Rural Africana* 26, 1974–1975: pp. 25–39.

Weissleder, Wolfgang. 'The Political Ecology of Amhara Domination'. Unpublished Ph.D. dissertation. University of Chicago, 1965.

Weldegebreil, Biniam. 'Traditional Medicine Practitioners of Addis Ababa: A Historical Account from Imperial Times to the

Present'. Unpublished B.A. thesis, Addis Ababa University. 1998.

Werner, David. *Where There Is No Doctor* (Amharic). Translated by Tena Abere. 2nd edition. Addis Ababa: Mega Publishing Agency, 2002.

WHO *see* World Health Organization.

Wogderes, Fikre Selassie. *We and the Revolution* (Amharic). Addis Ababa: Tsehay Printing Press, 2006 E.C.

Wolde Aregay, Merid. 'Traditional Medical Practice in a Historical Perspective'. 23rd Annual Dinner of the Ethiopian Medical Association. Addis Ababa, 1987.

Wolde Meskel, Mahatma Selassie. *Zekra Nagar: Recollection of Things Past* (Amharic). 2nd edition. Addis Ababa: Artistic Printing Press, 1962 E.C.

Wondmageghehu, Aymro and Joachim Motovu (eds.). *The Ethiopian Orthodox Church*. Addis Ababa: The Ethiopian Orthodox Mission, 1970.

Workineh, Habte Mariam, 'Teaching of the Ethiopian Orthodox Church on Matters Related to Health and Disease'. In *An Introduction to Health and Heath Education in Ethiopia*, compiled and edited by E. Fuller Torrey. Addis Ababa: Artistic Printers, 1967.

______. *Traditional Ethiopian Curriculum* (Amharic). Addis Ababa: Berhanena Selam Printing Press, 1962 E.C.

Workineh, Mekonnen. 'Developmental, Cultural and Political Contributions of the Ethiopian Orthodox Tewahdo Church to Ethiopia'. Unpublished B.Th. thesis. Holy Trinity Theological College, Addis Ababa, 1999.

World Health Organization, *Primary Health Care: Report of the International Conference on Primary Health Care*. Geneva: WHO, 1978.

______. 'Report of the Consultation on Approaches for Policy Development for Traditional Health Practitioners, Including Traditional Birth Attendants'. Geneva: WHO, 1985.

Worrell, W. H. 'Studien zum abessinischen Zauberwesen'. *ZA*, XXIII, 1909; XXIV, 1910; XXIX, 1914–1915.

Wright, W. *Catalogue of the Ethiopic Manuscripts in the British Museum Acquired Since the Year 1847*. London: Longmans & Co., 1877.

Ydlibi, May. *With Ethiopian Rulers: A Biography of Hasib Ydlibi*, Bahru Zewde (ed.). Addis Ababa: Addis Ababa University Press, 2006.

Yohannes, Wolde Giyorgis Wolde, *Agazi* (Amharic). Addis Ababa: Tesfa Gabra Selassie Printing Press, 1948 E.C.

Young, Allan. 'Medical Beliefs and Practices of Begemder Amhara'. Unpublished PhD. dissertation. University of Pennsylvania, 1970.

______. 'Why Amhara Get Kureynya: Sickness and Possession in an Ethiopian Zar Cult'. *American Anthropologist* 2(3), 1975: pp. 567–584.

______. 'Magic as a Quasi-Profession: The Organization of Magic and Magical Healing Among the Amhara'. *Ethnology* 14(3), 1975: pp. 245–265.

______. 'Externalizing and Internalizing Medical Beliefs: An Ethiopian Example'. *SSM* 10(3/4), 1976: pp. 147–156.

______. 'Order, Analogy and Efficacy in Ethiopian Medical Divination'. *Culture, Medicine and Psychiatry* 1(2), 1977: pp. 183–199.

______. 'The Practical Logic of Amhara Traditional Medicine'. In *African Therapeutic Systems*. Massachusetts: Crossroads Press, *c.* 1979.

______. 'The Relevance of Traditional Medical Culture to Modern Primary Health Care'. *Social Science and Medicine*, 17, 1983: pp. 1205–1211.

Zeleke, Afework (Alaqa). *Masehete Tibeb (Journal of Wisdom)* (Amharic). Addis Ababa: Ras Mekonnen Printing Press, 1926 E.C.

Zelleke, Knife-Rigbe, 'Bibliography of Ethiopic Hagiographical Traditions'. *JES*, 13(2), 1975: pp. 57–102.

Zeller, Diana. 'Traditional and Western Medicine in Buganda: Coexistence and Complement'. *Rural Africa*, 26, 1974/5: pp. 91–103.

Zewde, Bahru. *A History of Modern Ethiopia 1855–1974*. Addis Ababa: Addis Ababa University Press, 1991.

______. *Pioneers of Change in Ethiopia: Reformist Intellectuals of the Early Twentieth Century*. Addis Ababa: Addis Ababa University Press, 2002.

Archives

Dessie Municipality, Dessie. File no. መ 3-4; file no. m 3-5.

Dessie Regional Hospital, South Wallo. File no. 32/ሕ10/2.

Ministry of Information and National Guidance, A Communiqué entitled 'Religious Belief is an Enemy to the Revolution', n.d.

Ministry of Interior. Addis Ababa. File no. 2/93; File no. 4/2; File no. መ 5/27; File no. 22/22; File no. 29/63; File no. 37/50; File no. 41; File no. 131; File no. 131-መ 5; File no. 143- መ 5; File no. 161/1/402; File no. 161/402/7; File no. 331.

Ministry of Public Health. Addis Ababa. File no. ቀ-9 (hundreds of healers' personal files); File no. ወ-9; File no. ገሀ 23/45/13.

Public Records Office, F.O. 371, nos. 18028, 41498, 53458.

Wallo Provincial Health Department, Dessie. File no. ዴ-17; File no. ወ-6; File no. ወ-26.

Appendix: List of Oral Informants

Interviews were conducted with 63 cleric– and popular– or secular healers living in Addis Ababa, Bahir Dar, Debra Marqos, Debra Sina (Borana), Debra Tabor, Dalanta, Dessie, Gondar, Lalibela, Mahal Meda, Nafas Mewcha, Sayint, and Wadla (Kone). All informants were born, raised, and pursued their ecclesiastical and medico-magical education in the Amhara region, constituting North and South Gondar, East and West Gojjam, North and South Wallo and North Shewa. To correlate the oral data with informants, each informant is assigned a specific number and acknowledged in the footnote accordingly. This procedure has been applied to respect the anonymity of informants. Table A1 lists the informants, their ages, locations, place of interview and biographical information.

Table 1: Oral informant details

No.	Age	Date of Interview	Place of Interview	Remarks
1	60	27/01/2004 28/01/2004 29/01/2004	Bahir Dar (West Gojjam)	A school teacher with a background in ecclesiastical and church-based medical education
2	50	28/01/2004 –	Bahir Dar	A cleric–healer currently serving as Chairperson of

No.	Age	Date of Interview	Place of Interview	Remarks
		05/02/2004		the Amhara Regional Healers Association
3	62	Personal communication	Dessie (South Wallo)	A retired school teacher with advanced church education and a good recollection of church-affiliated medicine
4	69	Personal communication	Dessie	Full-time cleric–healer, a one-time Chairperson of the South Wallo Healers Association
5	56	05/02/04	Woldia (North Wallo)	Full-time cleric–healer from North Wallo, serving as itinerant healer together with a Muslim practitioner
6	66	06/02/04	Woldia (North Wallo)	A church-trained learned healer
7	78	Personal communication	Dessie	A learned clergy and a civil servant in the Ministry of Interior, now retired
8	68	30/12/2003	Mahal Meda (North Shewa)	A *dabtara* healer and 'book opener'
9	61	01/01/2004	Mahal Meda	Head of the Woreda Orthodox Church office
10	56	02/01/2004	Mahal Meda	A learned clergy working as a part-time cleric healer
11	77	30/01/2004	Bahir Dar	A learned cleric serving as a full-time healer
12	56	22/09/2003	Dalanta (North Wallo)	A learned healer, teaching a religious subject in a parish church
13	76 (?)	23/09/2003	Dalanta	A visually impaired and knowledgeable *qene* teacher
14	c.69	02/10/2003	Sayint (South Wallo)	*Qene* instructor with enormous recollection on the educational process of

No.	Age	Date of Interview	Place of Interview	Remarks
				the healing arts
15	70	01/10/2003	Mekane Selam (South Wallo)	A non-practitioner and *qene* instructor
16	57	10/05/2004	Dessie	An employee of a public transport firm and part-time medical practitioner
17	68	29/01/2004	Bahir Dar	A teacher in a *daber* church with a fair amount of knowledge on education *abinet*
18	73	18/10/2003 19/10/2003	Lalibela (North Wallo)	A cleric–healer/diviner of extensive learning and experience
19	51	20/10/2003	Lalibela	*Qene* teacher and part-time cleric–healer
20	81	21/10/2003 22/10/2003	Kone (North Wallo)	Former cleric–healer with enormous personal experiences as a student, and practitioner of herbal medicine and spirit invocation
21	72	01/10/2003	Debra Sina (South Wallo)	A clergyman with advanced ecclesiastical education and knowledge of the healing arts
22	75	10/11/2003	Debra Tabor (South Gondar)	A highly learned and full-time cleric–healer
23	56	03/11/2003	Nafas Mewcha (South Gondar)	An ecclesiastic and a part-time cleric–healer
24	61	03/01/2004 04/01/2004	Bahir Dar	A trained cleric who discontinued his religious duties to work as a full-time healer
25	79	06/11/03	Gondar	A cleric–healer with both

No.	Age	Date of Interview	Place of Interview	Remarks
			(North Gondar)	church and Western education, now a retired public servant.
26	52	15/02/2004	Debra Marqos (East Gojjam)	Full-time cleric–healer, and a former official of the provincial healers association
27	68	07/11/2003 08/11/2003	Gondar	An employee of a government office with long-time ecclesiastical studies and service as cleric–healer
28	41	09/11/2003	Gondar	A former student of an experienced cleric–healer, now a mechanic in a transport organisation
29	58	10/11/2003	Debra Tabor (South Gondar)	Full-time healer who picked up his medical knowledge from a number of Christian and Muslim practitioners.
30	50	10/11/2003 11/11/2003 12/11/2003	Debra Tabor	A cleric–healer who studied the healing arts from several cleric teachers, now Chairperson of the South Gondar Healers Association
31	63	11/12 /2003 12/11 /2003	Debra Tabor	A cleric–healer who claims to have inherited a very old medical manuscript from his uncle
32	40 (?)	20/12 /2003	Debra Marqos (East Gojjam)	A cleric–healer from Gondar who owned a clinic at Dessie for a brief period
33	57	18/11 /2004 21/01 /2005	Dessie	A handicapped *dabtara* with a good reputation of church-based healing techniques

No.	Age	Date of Interview	Place of Interview	Remarks
34	40	19/11 /2004 23/01/2005	Dessie	A son of a well-known *margeta* who inherited his father's medical manuscripts, currently working as a clerk in a parish church
35	58	31/01 /2004	Bahir Dar	A learned ecclesiastic who serves as a part-time healer
36	65	02/02 /2004	Bahir Dar	A full-time practitioner and an employee of the Bahir Dar Woreda Healers Association
37	63	02/01 /2004	Bahir Dar	A cleric–healer with several years of medical learning and healing service
38	52	01/02 /2004	Bahir Dar	A cleric–healer with additional skill in talismanic drawings
39	57	07/07/2004	Dessie	Part-time cleric–healer, serving as school guard
40	70	Personal communicati on	Addis Ababa	A *dabtara* working in the manuscript section of the IES library
41	62	18/05 /2004 19/05 /2004	Addis Ababa	Church-educated medical practitioner and Chairperson of the National Healers Association of Ethiopia
42	72	18/05 /2004	Addis Ababa	A person with a background in church education, and an official of the National Healers Association of Ethiopia
43	59	19/05 /2004	Addis Ababa	A church-educated healer and public relations officer of the National Healers Association of Ethiopia

No.	Age	Date of Interview	Place of Interview	Remarks
44	61	28/12 /2003	Nafas Mewcha (South Gondar)	A well-informed cleric–healer with many years of working experience
45	50	Personal communication	Dessie	A school teacher with a church background and part-time practitioner, now deceased.
46	63	26/04/2004	Sulula (South Wallo)	Herbalist–healer with long-time work experience
47	c.61	27/07/2004	Dessie	Herbalist–healer who treats skin diseases and a limited number of internal problems
48	63	28/07/2004	Dessie	Herbalist–healer specialising in skin diseases
49	67	03/08 /2004	Haiq (South Wallo)	A herbalist who treats a variety of internal and external illnesses
50	57	09/08/2004	Dessie	A literate Muslim herbalist–diviner with a high school education
51	60	03/08/2004	Haiq (South Wallo)	Herbalist–healer
52	68	03/10/2003	Debra Sina (South Wallo)	A learned ecclesiastic and cleric healer
53	60	11/08/2004	Dessie	Herbalist–healer
54	59	04/08/2004	Haiq	A herbalist, also commanding a limited knowledge of non-medication therapies
55	57	23/05/2004	Dessie	A long-time herbalist–healer
56	c.66	03/01/2004	Debra Berhan	Church-educated cleric–healer
57	84(?)	05/01/1991 07/01/1991	Dessie	The late *qene* instructor who had a remarkable

No.	Age	Date of Interview	Place of Interview	Remarks
				knowledge about church-based medicine and healing
58	53	Personal communications	Dessie	A trained psychiatrist nurse with good insight into the indigenous perspectives of mental problems
59	83	Personal communication	Dessie	A long-time resident of Dessie, and an oral historian of superb personal integrity and knowledge
60	72	Personal communication	Dessie	A former member of the armed forces with limited medical training, served as injectionist for very many years, now retired
61	70	Personal communication	Dessie	A health assistant in the Ministry of Education for more than three decades, became a full-time injectionist after his retirement
62	60	Personal communication	Dessie	Trained and served as a health assistant for many years and mustered a good knowledge of the injectionists. He had a private clinic until his death in 2005.
63	68	Personal communication	Dessie	A retired health assistant, still working as a dentist and injectionist

INDEX

A

B

C

D

E

F

G

H

I

J

K

L

M

N

U

V

W

Y

Z